NEURO PSYCHIATRY

MAUDSLEY PUBLICATIONS

WORKBOOK

MAUDSLEY PUBLICATIONS

ISBN number 0-9500289-8-3

PRODUCTION TEAM

AUTHOR & PRODUCER

Steve Church
Specialist Registrar in Neuropsychiatry, Institute of Psychiatry, London

DIRECTOR

Sir David Goldberg
Emeritus Professor of Psychiatry, Institute of Psychiatry, London

EDITORS

Anthony David
Professor of Cognitive Neuropsychiatry, Institute of Psychiatry and GKT School of Medicine, London

W Alwyn Lishman
Emeritus Professor of Neuropsychiatry, Institute of Psychiatry, London

SERIES CONSULTANTS

Colin Binnie
Professor of Neurophysiology, King's College Hospital, London

K Ray Chaudhuri
Consultant Neurologist, King's College Hospital, London

John M Dawson
Consultant Neuroradiologist,
Maudsley and King's College Hospital, London

Ian Everall
Professor of Neuropathology, Institute of Psychiatry, London

Simon Fleminger
Consultant Neuropsychiatrist, Maudsley Hospital, London

Laura Goldstein
Reader in Neuropsychology, Institute of Psychiatry, London

Michelle V. Lambert
Lecturer in Neuropsychiatry, Institute of Psychiatry
and GKT School of Medicine, London

Brian Toone
Consultant Neuropsychiatrist, Maudsley Hospital, London

CONTRIBUTORS

Peter Fenwick
Consultant Neuropsychiatrist, Maudsley Hospital, London

Simon Lovestone
Professor in Old Age Psychiatry and Psychopathology,
Institute of Psychiatry, London

John Mellors
Consultant Neuropsychiatrist, Maudsley Hospital, London

PROJECT ADVISOR

Dr D Bhugra
Senior Lecturer in Psychiatry, Institute of Psychiatry, London

CAMERAMAN AND VIDEO EDITOR

Terry O'Dowd
Media Support Unit, Maudsley Hospital, London

GRAPHIC DESIGNER

Alex Dionysiou
Medical Illustration, King's College, London

The course team would also like to thank the following:

VIDEO

Dr M Clark, *Medical Film & Video Library, The Wellcome Trust, London*
- for his assistance on video sources

Mr S Watts, *Manager, Media Support Unit, Maudsley Hospital, London*
- additional camera work

Dr JC Meadows, *Institute of Neurology, London*
- excerpt 1.3.2 taken from 'Disorders of language, reading and writing' 1974

Professor M Kopelman, *St Thomas' Hospital, London*
- excerpt 1.4.5

Mrs E Gascoigne and the National Society for Epilepsy
- excerpt 4.1.1 taken from their video ' Epileptic Seizures'

Dr J Dalton, *Janssen-Cilag Ltd*
- excerpt 4.1.2 taken from their video 'Fits and Faints'

Professor Satishcandra, *NIMHANS, Bangalore, India*
- excerpt 4.1.4

Dr F Besaq, *St Piers, Lingfield UK*
- excerpt 4.4

Professor MM Robertson, *The National Hospital, Queens Square, London*
- excerpt 7.2

Dr I Weber, *Knoll AG, D-67008, Germany*
- excerpt 7.3.1, 7.3.6 and 7.3.7 taken from the video 'Neuroeptic-Induced EPS' *(free tape available from Knoll AG)*

and all the patients who agreed to take part in this series

EDUCATIONAL ADVISOR

Professor J Grant
Professor of Education in Medicine, Open University
- for her helpful comments

EVALUATION CENTRES

The course materials have been evaluated on groups of psychiatrists (both trainees and senior academic staff) in the UK, Pakistan and India. Their comments on the content, style and timing of the modules have been an essential part of the development of the final package.

Dr R Gater and the Overseas Medical Graduates
Manchester University Department of Psychiatry, UK

Professor MH Mubbashar and the neuropsychiatrists from each region in Pakistan
Institute of Psychiatry and WHO Collaborating Centre, Rawalpindi, Pakistan

Professor RS Murthy and colleagues in his department
National Institute of Mental Health and Neurosciences, Bangalore, India

FUNDING

Psychiatric Research Trust,
Institute of Psychiatry, London

Charitable Funds,
South London and Maudsley Trust, London

C O N T E N T S

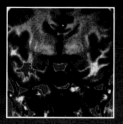

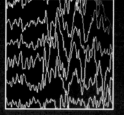

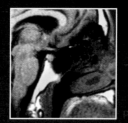

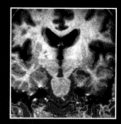

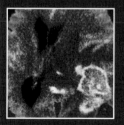

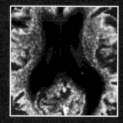

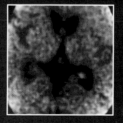

INTRODUCTION

WELCOME to the Maudsley neuropsychiatry modules. These modules cover topics relevant to psychiatrists and other medical professionals who wish to have further instruction in the diagnosis and management of neuropsychiatric conditions. The course comes out of a collaborative project at the South London and Maudsley Trust and the Institute of Psychiatry, London. The aim of the project has been to develop a teaching resource in neuropsychiatry that would be useful in many countries, either for self-paced learning or in small group teaching. This workbook and the accompanying videos are the outcome of the project.

Your workbook acts like a personal tutor, directing your study and focusing your efforts on what is most important to know. The content is modular; seven topics are chosen covering the general principles and key specific disorders of neuropsychiatry. Each module is divided into short sections to maintain interest and stimulate learning. Exercises are included to refresh your clinical skills and knowledge. The exercises are based around video excerpts of clinical interviews, case vignettes and results of specialist investigations. Feedback on the key learning points is given after each exercise; these points can act as prompts for further discussion when using the material in small group teaching or revision.

Selected references to your recommended reference textbook (*Organic Psychiatry 3rd edition* by W Alwyn Lishman) are given throughout which direct you to more detailed explanations and background theory.

The material is not exhaustive of the subject. What has been included has been selected for its perceived relevance and importance. Constraints of availability and the sensitive nature of showing video footage of actual patients has limited the scope of what can be shown. The majority of the individuals featuring in the video excerpts are either talking about past experiences from which they have recovered (with or without residual defects) or about the early symptoms of what will become a deteriorating condition. The aim is to highlight some aspects of the complexities of the subject whilst acknowledging that some issues concerning the clinical manifestations of acute organic reactions have not been featured. The focus is on adult neuropsychiatric disorders rather than on a comprehensive coverage of neurological clinical skills. There is no coverage of disorders specific to childhood and learning disabilities.

We hope that these modules will enhance your understanding of neuropsychiatry and that the learning experience will be both effective and enjoyable.

C O U R S E   S T R U C T U R E

If you have a workbook, two videos, a copy of the third edition of 'Organic Psychiatry' and something to write with, then you have the basics to get going. Print off a copy of the answer book from the disc provided and use this to write your answers on. Alternatively, simply write the answers down on a piece of paper. Work through the material at your own pace pausing between sections to reflect on the issues raised.

KEY

The following are the various graphic devices used throughout the workbook:

Video

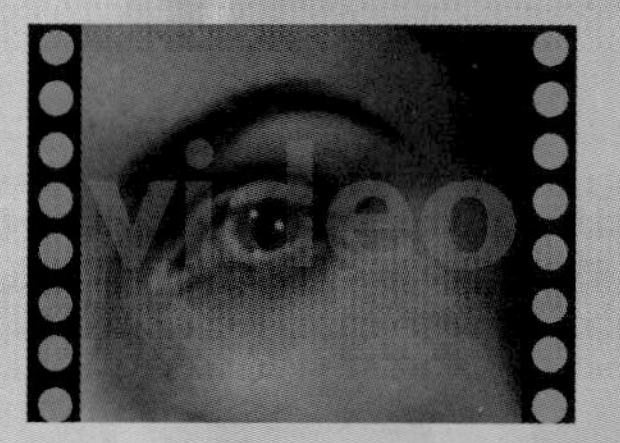

This graphic signifies that the exercise is based around either a single video excerpt or a series of excerpts (directions will be given in the text). When there are several excerpts associated with one exercise, pause the video between each, write an answer to the question given and then view the next excerpt. Timecodes are included on the video sleeve should you lose your place. Re-playing the video after reading the feedback will help reinforce the learning points. The aim has been to keep the excerpts short to avoid passive viewing!

Feedback

This signifies a feedback page to the exercise that you will have just completed; the key learning points raised by the questions are given. Try to think up your own answers before turning to the feedback in order to identify your strengths and weaknesses in the subject.

Reference

This graphic indicates some recommended reading from the textbook. Use this to study the background to the topics covered by the exercises. The modules broadly follow the main subject headings in Professor Lishman's *Organic Psychiatry 3rd edition*, starting with the principles of organic psychiatry and moving into the specific disorders. You will be directed to read selectively from this reference text.

MODULE I CONSULTANTS

Anthony David
W Alwyn Lishman

MODULE 1

Principles

CONTENTS

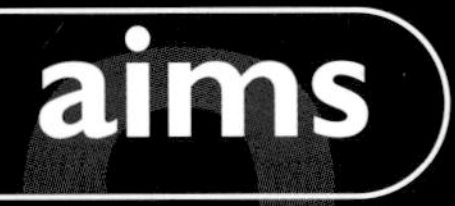

aims

This module aims to:

- introduce the principles of neuropsychiatry - the history and examination
- hightlight the usefulness of making a distinction between acute/chronic and focal/diffuse syndromes
- present the key focal cognitive syndromes of neuropsychiatric disorders

objectives

By the end of the module you should be able to:

- know a range of clinical tests used to screen for cognitive deficits
- be familiar with the areas of cognitive function typically affected by cerebral diseases
- know what syndromes are expected following lesions to different areas of the brain

PLAY THE VIDEO

Introduction 1.0

Excerpt 1.0 features Professor Lishman with Professor Goldberg, discussing the importance of eliciting a detailed history and tips on how to focus your examination. Eliciting accounts from others is emphasised.

Play the video from the beginning. Stop and return to this workbook when prompted

Introduction to chapter 1 and Nosology and the use of terms pp 3-9
The terminology of neuropsychiatry is complex. You may wish to read some background before proceeding. Further discussion is also found in the preface to 'Organic Psychiatry'.

1.1 - HISTORY

This section starts with a brief introduction to the basics of the history in neuropsychiatry. This includes the material you gain from the patient and informants and the sense that you can make of this by thinking in terms of syndromes of organic dysfunction. The history gives a longitudinal view of your patient's presentation. A minority of cases will give misleading presentations, especially in the early stages or where there is an abundance of non-organic features (i.e. in psychotic, conversion or factitious disorders). Focus on the mode of onset (and antecedent conditions) and the progression (the duration and fluctuations).

Subjective report

Establish your patient's own report of their experience; how they feel, what they see as the problem, how they regard their functioning to be impaired etc. This will give you an empathic understanding of their condition (the impact and meaning of their symptoms). Keep in mind that distortions may arise.

Distortions may arise from:

- degree of conscious awareness
- denial or minimisation
  (misleading account of the gravity of their difficulties)
- maximisation
  (increased awareness of deficits in depression)
- memory disorder and confabulation
- selective answering; answers dependant on state and context (e.g. offending)
- impairments to systems governing awareness of symptoms (may be symptom specific e.g. chorea)
- lack of insight

Objective report

It is vital to get a collateral history, to elicit observed symptoms as opposed to those felt. Early changes will be of a type more obvious to observers than to your patient (e.g. changes in alertness, memory, enthusiasms, habitual activities and attitudes). An informant can describe things that the patient never knew (because consciousness was impaired) and can describe changes in personality and cognitive functioning of which the patient is unaware.

Informants are not necessarily objective; distortions may also arise due to:

- deliberate falsifications
  (e.g. fabricating symptoms)
- denial
  (e.g. secondary to fear or a wish to protect the patient)
- ignorance of symptoms

⏩ ***History taking pp 94-5***
Read if necessary before moving on

SYNDROMES

Much of what you'll be studying in these modules involves identifying and understanding signs and symptoms. These can act as pointers to underlying disease processes and may cluster into syndromes which have localising value. There are two main syndrome distinctions that hold great importance in neuropsychiatry, namely;

ACUTE and/or CHRONIC

ACUTE

- abrupt onset with impairment of consciousness
- symptom pattern surprisingly constant;
  florid behavioural disturbance (with repetitive/purposeless/ stereotyped actions), labile affect, perceptual distortions and rich/intrusive fantasies (often persecutory and poorly elaborated)
- specific features depend on the rate of development, the intensity and the nature of the noxious agent
  e.g. infection, toxic, metabolic etc
- clinical picture is coloured by the personality and background of the patient
- majority reversible
  (but some progress to a chronic organic syndromes)

▸▸ ***clinical picture in acute organic reactions pp 9-13***

CHRONIC

- insidious onset with fluctuating level of consciousness, usually presenting with memory or performance failure
- blunting and dulling of psychic life; living deficiently in the real world
- majority are irreversible
  (but detection of those that aren't is a vital clinical skill)

▸▸ ***clinical picture in chronic organic reactions pp 13-16***

FOCAL and/or DIFFUSE

This distinction helps you localise pathology, discern treatable conditions and distinguish the relative contributions of impairment to resulting disability. Always contrast the preserved function with the impaired function.

FOCAL

- neurological signs are more reliable than psychiatric signs; e.g. hemiparesis, aphasia, unilateral anosmia and optic atrophy
- psychiatric manifestations tend to be isolated or standout against background of mild impairment
- localising e.g. Wernicke - Korsakoff's syndrome
- focal pathology can give rise to diffuse effects
  e.g. raised intracranial pressure due to intracranial tumour

DIFFUSE

- global deterioration of function due to diffuse neuropathology
  e.g. generalised atrophy, Lewy bodies or demylination

▸▸ ***clinical picture in focal cerebral disorder pp 16-20***

see also

▸▸ ***Differentiation pp 151-5***

This covers differentiation between these syndromes

LOCALISING SIGNS

First try an exercise that gets you to think about neuropsychiatric signs and syndromes, following either unilateral or bilateral lesions, which characterise cortical lobe dysfunction. Bear in mind the effects of cerebral dominance. Effects are greater with bilateral rather than unilateral lesions and those affecting the dominant rather than the non-dominant hemisphere.

Exercise 1.1

What neuropsychiatric features can accompany lesions to the following areas of the brain?

- Frontal lobe
- Temporal lobe
- Parietal lobe
- Occipital lobe
- Corpus callosum
- Diencephalon and brainstem

Answers will be given overleaf in the feedback, but write something down first before reading the answer. Further reading will be recommended at the end of the exercise that gives further information.

FRONTAL LOBE

Lesions may well be silent but the following signs can be found:

NEUROPSYCHIATRIC

- **Personality change**
  - profound change in disposition and temperament (more dramatic with bilateral lesions). Features include empty fatuous euphoria, social inappropraiteness (e.g. sexual disinhibition and overfamilarity), and problems with motivation and initiating actions.
    Two subtypes are described:
    - 'pseudodepressive' - akinesia (lateral frontal)
    - 'pseudopsychopathic - disinhibition (medialorbital)

- **Dysexecutive syndrome**
  - difficulties with planning, sequencing and executing tasks (but often in frontal lobe lesions IQ, memory and perception are preserved)

- **Broca's motor aphasia**
  (anterior dominant-inferior frontal hemisphere)

- **Loss of autonomy for individual actions**
  - **Perseveration** (motor/verbal)
    Inability to avoid repeating the last word or action, coupled with a failure to shift response pattern
  - **Motor impersistence**
    Patient is incapable of sustaining activities that they are capable of starting

- **Environmental dependancy**
  - **Magnetic syndrome**
    Grasp reflex coupled with 'sticky fixation' of hands which interferes with the execution of other movements
    » *pg 57*
  - **Utilisation behaviour** (orbital surface of frontal lobe)
    This is the pseudovoluntary (purposely but involuntary or automatic) use of objects present in surroundings or pathological dependancy on environmental stimuli.
    » *pg 106*

NEUROLOGICAL

- **Motor and premotor cortex signs**
  - contralateral spastic paresis; gait decompensation with truncal ataxia and postural change (precentral gyrus)
  - grasp reflex
  - sphincter incontinence (early - paracentral lobule)
  - supplementary motor area: acute paralysis of head and eye movements (turn to diseased side)

- **Ipsilateral optic atrophy** (optic nerve)

- **Anosmia** (olfactory nerve)

TEMPORAL LOBE

Most lesions are associated with a decrease in intellect (dominant > non-dominant), which contrasts with frontal lobe lesions. Non-dominant lesions often have a paucity of signs. The following signs can be found:

NEUROPSYCHIATRIC

- **Personality change**
  (limbic system)
  - similar to the change associated with frontal lesions but associated with intellectual and neurological deficits
  - emotional instability, aggression and paranoid states are common
  - depersonalisation and sexual disorders are less common (e.g. Kluver Bucy syndrome)

- **Amnesic syndromes**
  (bilateral medial involving hippocampus)
  - global amnesia with normal immediate recall
  - unilateral lesions give modality specific loss and rarely produce spontaneous complaint
  - lesions to the dominant hemisphere give verbal deficits
  - non-verbal memory (e.g. places, faces, music, drawing) is affected from non-dominant lesions

- **Wernicke's receptive aphasia**
  (superior temporal, dominant)
  - comprehension of language is affected

- **Prosopagnosia**
  (right inferior temporal gyrus)
  - impairment of facial recognition of known individuals

NEUROLOGICAL

- **Cortical deafness**
  (auditory cortex)

- **Contralateral upper quadrant homonymous hemianopsia**
  - single most important sign of deep lesion, affecting the optic radiation

- **Alexia and agraphia**
  (posterior)

PARIETAL LOBE

NEUROPSYCHIATIRC

- **Disorders of visuospatial integration**
  - visuospatial agnosia (including constructional apraxia)
  - astereognosis
  - toporaphical disorientation
    (these follow lesions of either lobe, being more common and severe with right side lesions)
- **Apraxias** (dominant)
- **Receptive dysphasias** (dominant)
- **Gerstmann's syndrome** (dominant)
  - finger agnosia, right/left disorientation, dyscalculia and dysgraphia
- **Body image disturbance** (non-dominant)
  - neglect (right supramarginal gyri)
  - anosognosia
- **Dyscalculia**

NEUROLOGICAL

- **Sensory disturbance** (anterior - primary sensory cortex)
  - contralateral sensory loss
    (asterognosis, agraphaesthesia and sensory extinction)
  - visual inattention
- **Contralateral lower quadrant hemianospia** (posterior)

OCCIPITAL LOBE

- **Visual hallucinations** (simple and complex)
- **Visual recognition difficulties**

CORPUS CALLOSAL

- **Callosal disconnection syndromes**
- **Intellectual deterioration** (anterior - severe and rapid)

DIENCEPHALIC and BRAINSTEM

- **Korsakoff-type amnesia** (especially deep midline)
- **Dementia**
  - rapid progression with intellectual deterioration secondary to hydrocephalus
- **Frontal type syndrome** (with better insight)
- **Other**
  - hypersomnia; emotional lability; stupor; akinetic mutism; pseudobulbar palsy; hypothalamic disorders

Further reference to localising signs are discussed in:

- ***Mental symptoms with tumours in different locations pp 222-31***
- ***Auras in epilepsy - initial focal onset of attack pp 249-52***

You may wish to read these before moving onto section 1.2

1.2 - EXAMINATION

The mental state examination gives you a cross-sectional view of your patient's condition. Your assessment at interview must be balanced against information of your patient's function in 'real life' settings. Further information can be gained by admission to hospital for a period of observation of behaviour (noting interactions and variability during the day), a thorough physical examination and specialist investigations (discussed in module 2).

This section focuses on the examination of the cognitive state, where bedside tests have evolved to screen for neuropsychiatric disorders. Some assessment of cognitive function should always constitute part of your general mental state examination.

▸▸ ***Physical examination pp 95-6***
▸▸ ***Mental state examination pp 96-8***
▸▸ ***Differential diagnosis pp 149-57***

You may wish to read further details of these areas

▸▸ ***Assessment of the cognitive state pp 98-107***
This reference provides the details of the tests you're about to see demonstrated. Try the exercise first without reading this reference; it is a more effective learning experience. You may wish to replay the excerpt a second time, after you've had time to review the feedback and further reading.

▶ PLAY THE VIDEO

Exercise 1.2

Excerpt 1.2 features Professor Lishman demonstrating the cognitive examination with a normal individual. The purpose of doing this is to introduce a test repertoire for examining cognitive dysfunction. The interview takes place at the Maudsley Hospital, London, on Friday 29th March 1999. This demonstration is fairly brief. If deficits had been encountered further questions and tests would have to be included to explore the deficits in greater detail. Several examples of such tests feature later in this module. Note also that several of the questions and tests would need to be adapted when examining a patient in a country other than the UK.

Answer question 1.2.1 after you have seen the demonstartion. Feedback is given over the next three pages.

1.2.1

What tests are used to examine the following areas?

- Orientation
- Concentration and Attention
- Language
- Memory
- Visuospatial function
- 'Frontal' function
- Body image and right/left orientation

FEED BACK

Professor Lishman starts by putting Martin at ease. This is a vital first step because the tests are anxiety provoking. He then moves on to test the following:

ORIENTATION

- **Time/Place/Person**
  Disorientation is a key indication of cerebral dysfunction, reflecting alterations in the level of consciousness. Time disorientation is regarded as the hallmark of acute organic reactions.

CONCENTRATION and ATTENTION

- **Reciting backwards** e.g. reverse days of the week
- **Serial 7's** - counting down from 100 in subtractions of 7
- **Digit span recall - forwards and backwards**
  (average 7 forward)
  These test alertness and the capacity to control information processing in the brain. Along with tests for orientation, these are a means of evaluating your patients level of conscious awareness; an assessment which is a priority given that it affects all other tests.

LANGUAGE

Handedness

Professor Lishman first clarifies whether Martin is left or right handed as >95% of right-handers and the majority of left-handers have relative language dominance in the left hemisphere. Having noted that motor aspects of speech are apparently intact, he next examines:

Repetition

- **"West Register St"** and **"no ifs, ands or buts"**
  These test for dysarthria and the intactness of the connections between the input and output of speech.

Comprehension

- **Response to simple instructions**
  - point correctly on command (e.g. plant and lamp)
  - carry out simple orders on request
    (e.g. pick up an object/show tongue)

- **Response to complex instructions**
  - tear paper into three pieces (Marie's 3 paper test)

Word finding

- **Name both common and uncommon objects**
  - (e.g. parts of a wrist watch, and other objects in the room)
    This tests for nominal dysphasia (the reduced capacity to retrieve words used in everyday speech) which may be the only language disturbance. Note circumlocutions used to cover this deficit.

Reading

- **Observe for content errors**
  (also dysarthria and dysprosody)

Writing

- **Test ability to write spontaneously**
  Examine written productions for substitutions, perseverations, spelling errors and letter reversals. Note that asking a patient to write something of what they've just read (e.g. news item) also further tests their comprehension.

MEMORY

NB Test verbal and non-verbal memory re-call

- **Immediate memory span** (or `ultra-short-term-memory')
  - digit repetition (tested previously)

- **Recent events**
  - recall of the temporal sequence of events (e.g. the events of the interview)

- **New learning**
  - **Name and address**
    Ask for immediate reproduction and record the answer verbatim (not shown on tape) - *repeat if necessary*
    Test retrieval 3-5 minutes later after interposing other cognitive tests, and again record the answer verbatim
  - **Babcock Sentence**
    e.g.:"One thing a nation needs to become rich and great is a large secure supply of wood"
    - ask your patient to repeat a sentence appropriate to their intellectual level. Test the number of repetitions necessary for the accurate reproduction.
      (Three repetitions of such a sentence should allow word perfect reproduction in a patient of average intelligence)

- **General Information**
  - semantic (conceptual) memory
    e.g. names of key personalities, well-known dates, places and events both distant and current
  - episodic (personal) memory -
    matters unique to the individual
    e.g. what they ate for breakfast

NOTE

In this demonstration Martin is then asked to perform addition, subtraction, multiplication, division; these test for dyscalculia and are also being used as a distracting activity prior to testing for delayed recall (name and address).

FEED BACK

VISUOSPATIAL

- **Distance estimation between objects** - test proportions
- **Copy a diagram** - tests constructional ability/non-verbal memory
- **Freehand drawing** - test for neglect and aphasia
  e.g. drawing a clock face with numbers

NOTE
Your patient is unlikely to draw attention to any non-verbal deficits; if you don't test for them, the deficits will remain concealed. Note for neglect of visual space and perseverations

FRONTAL LOBE

- **Verbal Fluency** - e.g. words beginning with the letter 'F'
  (FAS test - 10 words per letter in one minute is the average)
- **Luria's motor tests** for sequencing and perseveration
- **Abstract thinking and conceptualisation**
  - proverbs
    e.g. "People in glass houses shouldn't throw stones"
  - difference between concepts
    e.g. child and dwarf
- **Cognitive Estimates Test**
  e.g. largest object in a household room

NOTE
Note how Professor Lishman takes the opportunity, after a few minutes, to assess non-verbal memory by asking for reproduction of the shapes drawn.

BODY IMAGE and RIGHT-LEFT ORIENTATION

- **Name and point** to various parts of the body (spatial orientation to self and object)

▸▸ ***Assessment of the cognitive state pp 98 - 107***
Study further details on this issue before moving on

NOTE - Intelligence
There is an important difference between intelligence as measured by clinical tests and psychometry and 'real-life' intelligence (i.e. dealing with the complexities of the outside world). These tests provide information in addition to that gleaned in the history, against which to make a clinical judgement of generalised intellectual impairment. Always interpret these tests in terms of your patient's education and cultural background. Psychometric (formal) tests also allow a reliable baseline to be established against which decline can be measured.

FOCAL COGNITIVE SYNDROMES

The remaining units (1.3-1.8) in this module look at each function tested for in Professor Lishman's video. Clinical examples are given using tests you've just seen demonstrated. You will then be asked to try and identify the dysfunction(s) shown. The divisions are artificial given the dynamic interaction between brain and mental processes; alterations in one sphere often lead to abnormalities in other areas. The important concept to remember is that each function has localising value.

1.3 - LANGUAGE

Efficient communication of information requires symbols. Language is the ability to code and interpret those symbols. It relates closely to thought and has four main components;

- **semantic** (symbolic meaning of words)
- **syntactic** (relational aspects of language involving ordering to produce grammatically correct expression)
- **prosodic** (melody, inflection, rhyme and timbre that convey emotional meaning)
- **gestural** (movement and expression used to enhance general meaning)

Dysphasia (or aphasia) is the name given to abnormalities of language. Assessing for dysphasia is crucial before proceeding with further cognitive testing. There is either a defective understanding of speech/writing or a defective production of speech/writing. The main syndromes are: primary sensory dysphasia (fluent); primary motor dysphasia (non-fluent); nominal dysphasia (naming); conduction aphasia (loss of repetition); and transcortical dysphasia (motor and sensory language disorder with preserved repetition). 'Pure' syndromes are also described but are rare.

▸▸ ***Clinical syndrome of language impairment pp 49-55***
You may wish to read further details before proceeding

PLAY THE VIDEO

Exercise 1.3

The following video sequence starts with a further demonstration from Professor Lishman (excerpt 1.3.1) and then shows you a range of manifestations of language dysfunctions seen clinically (excerpt 1.3.2-8).

Watch each excerpt separately, pausing between each to write down an answer. Over the page you will find feedback, but don't turn over until you've watched each excerpt.

1.3.1 Extending the assessment of language

What aspect of language function is tested
(think why the test may be important)

Excerpts 1.3.2- 1.3.8

What language abnormalities are being demonstrated in each excerpt?
(Hint: all the excerpts show different language dysfunction)

1.3.2 Elderly man recounting a story
1.3.3 Woman's orientation being examined
1.3.4 Man repeating a tongue twister
1.3.5 Woman naming common objects and defining words
1.3.6 Man being asked to read the word 'hutch'
1.3.7 Young man being asked to count to ten
1.3.8 Old man talking about a strike at work

1.3.1

- **Detailed testing of comprehension, including syntax**
  Syntax concerns the grammatical relationship between words taking account of their order in a sentence. The key here is the ability to comprehend the serial relationship of the request ("Place.."/"Pick up…put…..touch"). This test is useful in detecting otherwise silent abnormalities of language.

1.3.2

- **Wernicke's receptive/sensory dysphasia - fluent**
  Note how the speech is fluent with normal syntax but lack of meaningful content, reflecting a defective appreciation of the meaning of words. (Δ dementia)

1.3.3

- **Broca's expressive/motor dysphasia - non-fluent**
  Here the deficit lies in the effector side of speech altering the mechanisms by which words are chosen and articulated and sentences constructed. Circumlocution (and time disorientation) is evident, shown by the patient not being able to find the correct word and therefore talking around the point using gestures. (Δ early onset dementia)

1.3.4

- **Conduction dysphasia**
  The patient fails to repeat the sentence given, despite otherwise being able to speak, suggesting a disconnection between Broca's and Wernicke's areas. Note how he rushes into the task, quickly gives up and appears frustrated and upset (catastrophic reaction). (Δ focal dementia)

1.3.5

- **Nominal Dysphasia**
  The principal difficulty here lies in evoking names at will; note how it improves with cueing (giving 3 alternatives) and that the patient retains the knowledge of what each object is used for (which contrasts with visual object agnosia and semantic dementia). The fact that she can use a pen when asked shows she is not suffering from apraxia. This is one of the commonest manifestation of dysphasia. (Δ post - encephalitis)

1.3.6

- **Pure Word-blindness**
  The condition is incompletely demonstrated but the main difficulty in this disorder lies in understanding what's read. The patient is unable to recognise the language values of the visual patterns which make up whole words and hence can't say 'hutch'. There is no disturbance of the symbolic function of the words themselves presented in other modalities or in language output. This condition is believed to reflect a disconnection of visual input from language processing. (Δ stroke)

1.3.7

- **Dysarthria and dysphonia**
  The patient comprehends and executes the command. His difficulty lies in the articulation, not production, of words. (Δ athetoid cerebral palsy)

1.3.8

- **Neologisms**
  The words 'clausal'/sedential' are not recognised in English. The condition doesn't fit into a neurological classification. The speech is pedantic and concerned with detail. The empty stereotyped phrases reflect the disordered thought processes. (Δ schizophrenia)

» ***Clinical syndrome of language impairment pp 49-55***
See also pg 39-48 for reference then when you ready move on to the next section

1.4 - MEMORY

Amnesia is the name given for acquired memory dysfunction. There is an abonormality in registering, storing, recalling or recognising information and events. Focal amnesic states, from discrete lesions, can occur with relative preservation of other cognitive functions, whilst diffuse amnesic states occur with other cognitive dysfunction. All are qualitatively different from psychogenic amnesias. Memory failure is a particularly sensitive indicator of cerebral dysfunction. Remember that your patient may have deficits in explicit memory, with difficulty in conscious recollection, yet retain implicit (procedural/skills) knowledge. For example, they may be able to find their way around familiar surroundings but be unable to recollect (describe) their route.

▸▸ ***Clinical picture in amnesia pp 28-34***
Read further details in you need to before proceeding

▶ PLAY THE VIDEO

Exercise 1.4

The video sequence in this exercise again starts with a demonstation of an extension to the cognitive examination, this time evaluating memory(excerpt 1.4.1). Excerpts 1.4.2-5 cover selected examples of amnesic syndromes.

Watch each excerpt separately, writing an answer for the question given.

1.4.1 Alternative to the name and address test

What test of memory is being shown?
(Think also of a simpler version of this test)

Excerpts 1.4.2 - 1.4.4

What abnormality of memory is demonstrated in the each of the following ?

1.4.2 Young man describing recent difficulties
1.4.3 Elderly man recollecting
1.4.4 Middle aged man repeating a story

1.4.5 Man interviewed about recent events

The man in this excerpt has suffered a documented Wernicke's encephalopathy. He is being interviewed two months after the event. The interview takes place on a Monday in November 1991.

What features of the Korsakoff's syndrome are demonstrated and what other features would you like to elicit?

1.4.1

- **Recall (paired association) - free and cued**
  Storage is tested by giving verbal cues when spontaneous recall fails; a retrieval deficit is suggested if the patient's performance improves. A simpler test is of 3 word recall, each word being categorically different e.g. flower, colour and town. Information processing is also being tested, as recall is facilitated by thinking of semantic links. These tests are especially valuable with anxious or disturbed patients.

1.4.2

- **Resolving amnesia**
  The patient describes impairments in acquiring (learning) new information and recalling recent events.
  (Δ haemorrhage from an arteriovenous malformation)
  ▸▸ ***Amnesic syndrome following subarachnoid bleed pp 392-6***

1.4.3

- **Retrieval deficits from the remote past**
  (Δ post encephalitis)

1.4.4

- **Confabulation** (and drifting into irrelevant material)
  The falsification of memory occurring in clear consciousness in association with an organically derived amnesia. It may be:
  - provoked (momentary/fleeting) - evident only on probing, as with this example
  - spontaneous (sustained/grandiose) - evident in general conversation.

  (Δ acute aftermath of a traumatic brain injury)
  ▸▸ ***Confabulation pp 30-1***

1.4.5

Features of Korsakoff's syndrome demonstarted:

- **Impairment of recall**
  e.g. reasons for admission/name of prime minister and date of general election
- **Preserved alertness and language**
- **Time disorientation;** faulty judgement of passage of time

Further features to elicit:

- **Confirm impaiment of new learning by formal testing**
- **Seek to establish lengthy retrograde amnesia**
- **Confirm other cognitive functions are substantially intact** i.e. establish a disproportionate memory loss using psychometry
  Korsakoff's syndrome is a classic example of a focal persistent amnesic syndrome, where memory and new learning are affected out of proportion to other cognitive functions in an otherwise alert and responsive patient. Confabulation is not invariably found.
  ▸▸ ***Wernicke's encephalopathy and Korsakoff's syndrome pp 577-85***
  ▸▸ ***Korsakoff's syndrome in alcoholic dementia pg 603***

See also:

▸▸ ***Hypothalamic and diencephalic systems pp 25-7***
▸▸ ***Clinical picture in amnesia pp 28-34***
▸▸ ***Unresolved problems in amnesic states pp34-9***
▸▸ ***Alcoholic blackouts pp 595-7***
▸▸ ***Transient global amnesia pp 413-7***

1.5 - VISUOSPATIAL FUNCTION

In order for sensations to be fully appreciated and consciously recognised they have to be perceived, discriminated and associated with existing knowledge. Stimuli have to be processed ('apperception') to form a conscious perception of something. These conscious elements then need to be associated (linked) with other elements (e.g. memory traces) which give them meaning. Abnormality in this higher level process leads to agnosia, a disorder of perceptual recognition (not attributed to a primary sensory deficit or general intellectual impairment). Thus perceptual disorders can be subdivided into apperceptive and associative agnosias. They are rare and complex disorders. What you need to keep in mind is that all modalities may be affected but visuospatial problems are more common.

➧ ***Agnosia and related defects of perception pp 58-65***
If you need to, read more about these complex disorders before tackling the exercise

▶ P L A Y   T H E   V I D E O

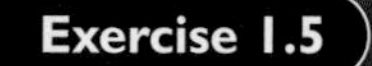

Exercise 1.5

Two excerpts feature here; they cover two key areas of perceptual disturbance.
Write down your answer to each example before turning to the feedback.

1.5.1 Right handed woman asked to copy a clock and flower. She drew the right hand image of each pair:

What condition do you think she has ?

1.5.2 A man describing resolving problems

What abnormalities does he describe ?

FEED BACK

1.5.1

- **Visuospatial agnosia and hemineglect**
  - visual neglect shown by omissions in images copied i.e. the numbers of the clock are crowded onto the right hand side, and one half of the flower is missing (Δ right hemisphere stroke with resulting in a left-sided hemiplegia)

1.5.2

- **Prosopagnosia** (improving)
  - prosopagnosia is the inability to recognise faces
- **Topographical disorientation**
  (Δ encephalitis)

NOTE

Firm indications of a pure agnosic problem will often be obtained by finding the subject retains knowledge about the object despite the fact that the object cannot be identified through one sensory modality (e.g. not being able to describe a telephone, but naturally answering it if it rings)

Other visual perceptual abnormalities to assess include;

- **Visual object agnosia** (visual recognition failure)
  - describe an object

  The patient fails to identify the objects by sight and fails to name them; ie she is unable to get the meaning of the object purely by looking at them. It is essential to exclude impairments of primary perception as the cause of failure on a test (such as impaired visual acuity, field defects, or deafness)
- **colour anomia** (inability to name colours)
  - test by asking patient to name colours and to group objects according to their colour

Rarer agnostic difficulties include:

- **Auditory agnosia**
  - assessed when testing comprehension of speech
- **Tactile agnosia or Astereognosis**
  - test by asking patient to identify objects by touch with the eyes closed, each side being tested separately
- **Topographagnosia**
  - test by identifying location on a map
- **Simultanagnosia**
  - ask patient to describe multiple objects in a scene

▸▸ ***Agnosia and related defects of perception pp 58-65***
You may wish to re-read more about these complex disorders before moving on

1.6 - PRAXIS

The previous section dealt with high level disorders of perception. Here we look at high level motor abnormalities; the dyspraxias. Apraxia is the inability to carry out learned, voluntary movements (or movement complexes) which cannot be accounted for by paresis, inco-ordination or sensory loss. It's rarely seen without dysphasia, except in the case of constructional dyspraxia. This section highlights tests that screen for two features of the disorder.

▸▸ ***Apraxia (dyspraxia) and related executive disorders pp 55-8***

You may wish to refer to these pages during the next exercise

PLAY THE VIDEO

Exercise 1.6

Excerpt 1.6 shows tests for dyspraxia

Write down an answer to the question below after you've seen the excerpt. Feedback is given over the page but try answering the question before looking

1.6.1

What 2 types of apraxia are being assessed by these tests ?

(describe how these are tested)

video

1.6.1

- **Ideomotor apraxia**
  - tested by the ability to imitate postures and make-believe movements (e.g. wave goodbye)

  Ideomotor apraxia is the inability to carry out simple co-ordinated movement sequences on command, despite being able to carry out these actions spontaneously. The individual cannot, at will, start a movement.

- **Ideational apraxia**
  - (e.g. fold a letter and put it in an envelope)

  Ideational apraxia is the inability to carry out a planned complex co-ordinated sequence, despite demonstrating an ability to carry out each individual component. The individual cannot, at will, guide a series of consecutive movements in a the correct spatial/temporal sequence (ideational apraxia), even though the same muscles can be used and analogous move-ments performed in other contexts. Ideational apraxia is nearly always due to bilateral damage, associated with diffuse neuropathology, and is often accompanied by dysphasia and a decline in intellectual ability.

NOTE

It is vital to exclude simple unwillingness to co-operate

Other apraxias include:

- **Limb kinetic**
- **Whole body**
  - test by commanding to stand up / turn around
- **Dressing**
  - note for muddling clothes and difficulty dressing

▸▸ ***Apraxia (dyspraxia) and related executive disorders pp 55-8***

You may wish to re-read these pages before moving on

1.7 - FRONTAL LOBE FUNCTION

Evidence of frontal lobe damage would have been suggested by a history of behavioural disturbance (e.g. disinhibition, apathy, poor social awareness etc), personality change and 'executive dysfunction' (e.g. disturbance to planning and monitoring goal-directed behaviours). The exercise in this section highlights some of the bedside tests employed to further evaluate this damage. In clinical practice, these need to be supplemented by more detailed psychometric assessment.

▸▸ ***Frontal lobe syndrome pp76-80***
You may wish to read further details before attempting this exercise

▶ PLAY THE VIDEO

Exercise 1.7

Two excerpts feature in this exercise. Excerpt 1.7.1 is a brief interview with a woman who displays several features of frontal lobe dysfunction but also highlights an important aspect of differentiating disorders. Excerpt 1.7.2 highlights other effects of frontal lobe damage.

Watch each excerpt separately, writing an answer for each question. Feedback is given over the page but try answering each question before looking.

1.7.1 An elderly woman being tested on two separate occasions; before and after treatment

What abnormalities of frontal lobe function are demonstrated and what might account for her different presentation the second time you see her?

1.7.2 A man being asked the meaning of a phrase

What frontal test is being shown and what does it highlight?

FEED BACK

1.7.1

Δ The woman in this case had a frontal meningioma.
On the first occasion you see her (pre-treatment), she displays the following abnormalities, characteristic of frontal lobe dysfunction:

- **Impaired Verbal Fluency**
- **Irritability**
- **Disinhibited social behaviour**

The second occasion (post-treatment) shows the remarkable post operative improvement;the patient has regained a more balanced composure and engages in the tests with willingness and humour. But verbal fluency remains poor. This case highlights the importance of identifying reversible conditions.

1.7.2

- **Abstract thinking** tested with proverb interpretation i.e. 'people in glass houses'
The patient shows 'literal/concrete thinking'; even with encouragement, he can't generalise.

(Δ Traumatic brain injury secondary to severe assault)

see also

- ***Frontal lobe test pp 105-6***
- ***Organic personality change pp 7-8***

1.8 - BODY IMAGE

Body image (or 'schema') is the subjective model of the body against which changes can be appreciated. Neuropsychiatric body image disturbance can be divided into unilateral or bilateral dysfunction. This section takes an excerpt from a clinical interview to highlight an unusual condition.

▸▸ ***Disorders of body image pp 67-76***
This reference provides further details, which you may wish to read before the exercise

PLAY THE VIDEO

Exercise 1.8

1.8.1 Woman being asked about her left hand

Watch the next excerpt of the woman you saw earlier who developed left hemiparesis following a stroke two months before the recording was made. Cognitive testing has already established that she is orientated, with normal language and memory. She is right handed and is shown discussing her left arm.

What clinical condition does she describe and what features of this condition are highlighted?

1.8.1

- **Anosognosia** - lack of awareness or denial of abnormality
  This is an example of a unilateral disturbance, often occuring with unilateral inattention and neglect. It typically follows pathology in the right hemisphere more than the left, hence presenting more often with left sided neglect. Commonly anosognosia is merely a transient state and recedes along with the initial clouding of consciousness. However it may persist and become more floridly developed with obstinate denial or bizarre elaboration on a delusional basis (as is the case here).

Features displayed include:

- **Emotional indifference 'anosodiaphoria'**
  The patient sits calmly in her wheelchair, showing no apparent distress to her paralysed arm.
- **Denial**
  When asked to touch the examiner's finger, she claims to have carried this through, despite not moving her left side. This denial reflects severe anosognosia. She had no doubt that she is right. That she can touch her left hand with her right shows there is no personal neglect or hemisomatoagnosia. Patients often have a dim awareness of their deficit and aim to cover it up or deflect attention to another topic.
- **Delusions: `somatoparaphrenia'**
  This patient insists that the paralysed limb does not belong to her and attributes it to someone else ("I think it's a man's arm")
  Additional features can include:
  - belief that limb has an existence of its own (`personification')
  - feelings of anger or hatred expressed towards the limb (`misoplegia')

Bilateral disturbance of body image is suggested by:

- **Right-Left disorientation**
- **Autotopagnosia** the inability to recognsise, name or point to various parts of the body.

M1 SUMMARY

We've come to the end of module one, having covered a vast area in a short space of time. You may wish to consolidate the key learning points of focal cortical dysfunction before taking a look at the specific disorders in which they feature (modules 3-7).

MODULE 2 CONSULTANTS

EEG: Colin Binnie
Neuroimaging: John Dawson
Psychometry: Laura Goldstein

MODULE 2

Investigations

CONTENTS

aims

This module aims to:

- introduce three specialist investigations
- highlight the uses and limitations of these investigations in neuropsychiatry
- provide a basis for interpreting the results in different clinical contexts

objectives

By the end of this module you should be able to:

- understand the basics of encephalography (EEG) and be able to identify abnormal phenomenon on EEG traces
- understand the basics of neuroimaging and be able to identify cerebral abnormalities using structural imaging techniques
- know the range of psychometric tests available and appreciate their uses in evaluating neuropsychiatric conditions

PLAY THE VIDEO

Introduction 2.0

Excerpt 2.0 features Professor David with Professor Goldberg, discussing the uses and indications of specialist investigations in neuropsychiatry. The investigative techniques aide the process of localisation of neuropathology, establish baselines and further guide your clinical management.

▸▸ *Ancillary investigations pp 126-7 and Lumbar puncture pp 133-4*

This reference covers routine investigations (e.g. serological and urine tests) used to screen for systemic causes of organic psychiatric disorders (e.g. 'Endocrine Diseases and metabolic disorders' and 'Toxic disorders' etc). Details of these issues will not be further discussed in this module.

2.1 - ELECTROENCEPHALOGRAPHY (EEG)

The EEG is a tracing; a record of the sychronous neural activity from scalp electrodes. It is an epiphenomenon reflecting the summated post-synaptic potentials of cortical neurones when they're 'idling' and not processing information. In this state their activity is synchronous. When transmitting and processing information, their activity becomes asynchronous (or de-synchronised). The main advantage of EEG is that it is a non-invasive means of determining the physiological or functional state of the brain, as opposed to its anatomical status. It can suggest abnormal function when imaging indicates normal gross structure. It's main limitation is that not it's not specifically diagnostic.

▸▸ ***Electroencephalography pp 127-33***
If you need to consult these pages whilst working through this section

▶ PLAY THE VIDEO

Introduction 2.1

Excerpt 2.1 features Professor Binnie with Professor Goldberg, discussing the theory and practicalities of EEG recordings; including the use of monitoring - prolonged recording with telemetry. Professor Binnie then takes you through the normal and abnormal findings on EEG, and procedures used to activate the patient (see below). The excerpt concludes with the clinical indications for EEG.

Normal findings:
- power spectrum/freguency bands
- normal waking adult
- drowsiness and sleep
- age-related changes

Abnormal phenomenon:
- asymmetry and slowing (e.g. Alzheimer's)
- 'epileptiform activity'
- 'spikes', 'sharp waves' and 'spike and wave'

Activation procedures:
- hyperventilation
- photic stimulation
- sleep

Watch the excerpt and stop when prompted. There is no exercise around this piece. Read through the next few pages which orientates you to features of the EEG. When you're ready, have a go at exercise 2.1

RECORDING VARIABLES: amplitude and frequency

Two main features of EEG recordings are the amplitude and frequency. Understanding the factors that cause these variables to alter will help you distinguish between normal and abnormal findings.

■ **Amplitude** - function of both activity and synchrony

e.g. a recording of low amplitude may be due to either hightened arousal, anxiety or during a difficult cognitive task OR secondary to lack of neural activity (e.g. terminal stages of dementia, coma etc).

■ **Frequency** - ongoing activity and episodic/transient events

Ongoing activity - 4 main frequency bands

Delta <4/sec (4Hz)

- diffuse distribution in children and sleeping adults (preponderant component in deep sleep)
- abnormal in awake adults

Theta 4 - <8/sec (Hz)

- temporal dominance; normal in children and adolescents and present in small amounts in most of the normal population

Alpha 8 - <14 /sec (Hz)

- dominant rhythm in parietoccipital, increasing with eye closure, relaxation (alpha bursts) and absence of sensory stimuli
- decreasing with age, increasing arousal and cognitive processing

Beta >14/sec (Hz)

- frontocentral dominance (inversely proportional to alpha).
- most prominent EEG component with eyes open
- increased with anxiety, alcohol and drugs

Episodic and transient events

- **Spikes** <80 msec, high amplitude
- **Sharp waves** 80 - 200 msec
- **Spike and wave complexes** short, high amplitude
- **Slow waves** >200 msec
- **Sleep spindles** frontal bursts at 10 - 14/sec
- **K complexes** sharp and slow waves at the vertex, related to arousal
- **Parietal-occipital sharp transients of sleep (POSTS)** posterior sharp waves
- **'Rhythms at a distance'** rhythmic bifrontal slow activity ('Frontal intermittent rhythmic delta activity' or FIRDA) and posterior slow waves

MONTAGES (WIRING DIAGRAMS)

There is a standard system for electrode placement, which uses anatomical landmarks. Several settings may be adopted, depending on the clinical condition in question. The following diagrams highlight the main placements used; the numbering on the left hand side of the EEG recording links with the number on the montage. These montages will feature as thumbnails in exercise 2.1 to help you link abnormal findings with the likely brain region.

Bipolar

Recordings made from this set-up comprise local potential gradients between adjacent electrodes

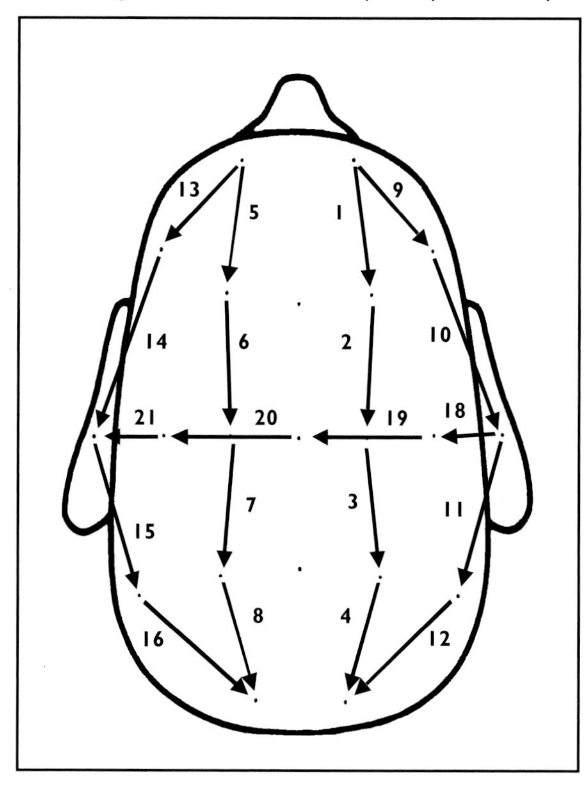

Double banana

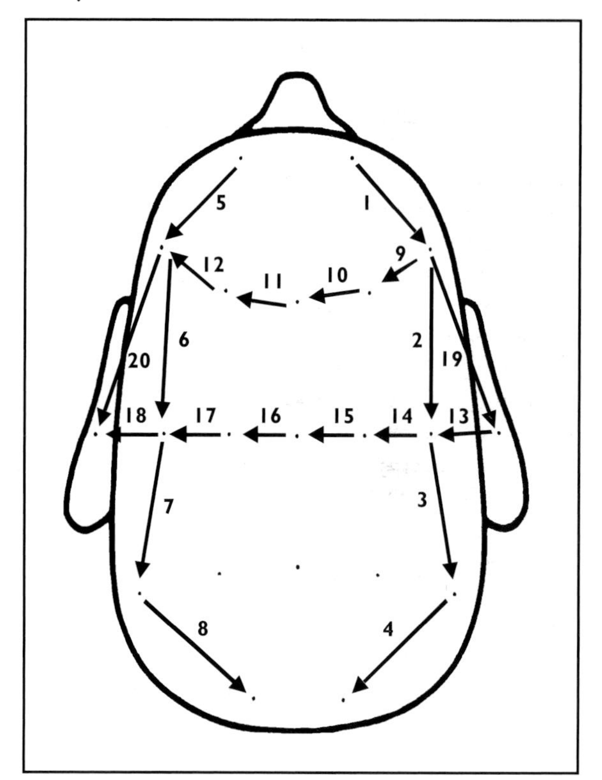

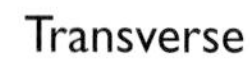

Transverse

Common average reference

Record voltage with respect to the average of the whole electrode array

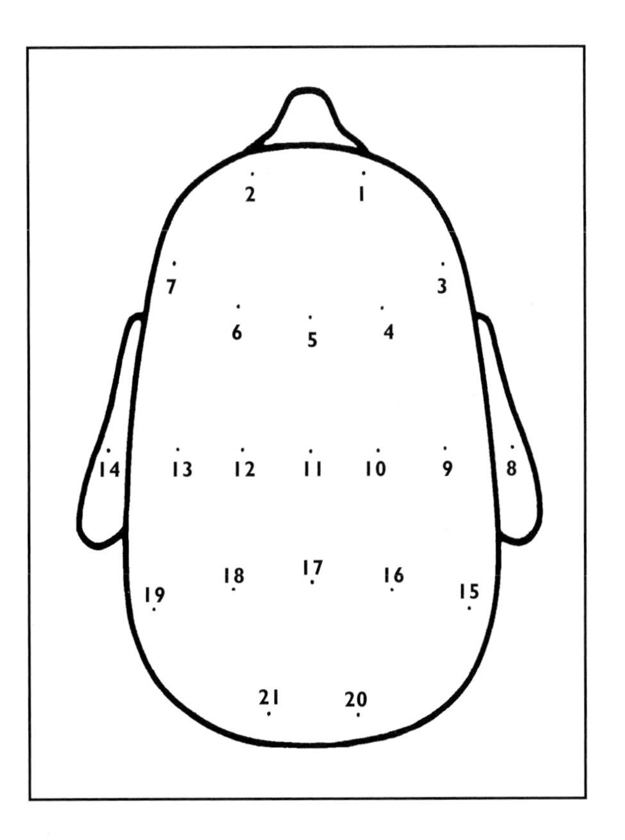

Photic stimulation

These record potential gradients (like bipolar) and are used in photic activation studies

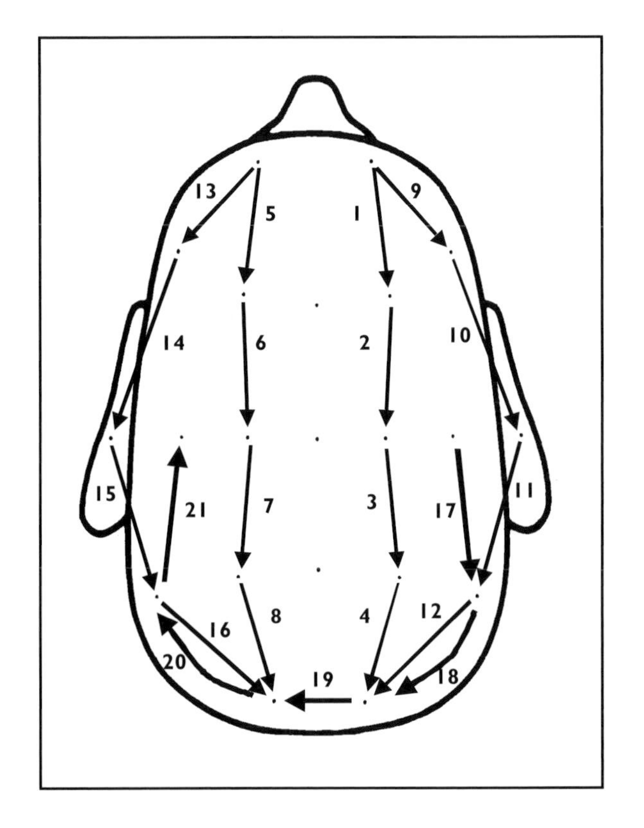

Exercise 2.1

This exercise starts by encouraging you to reflect on the clinical usefulness of EEG (2.1.1). This is followed by several examples of EEG recordings (2.1.2-8); the aim with these is to help you to identify important features. Note that diffuse lesions produce rhythmic slowing and focal lesions produce local arrhythmias.

Also, several factors can influence the recording, including:

- **Physical factors**
  Interference (physical/electrical) and biological artifact (muscle activity/eye-movement) can obscure the tracing

- **Physiological variables**
  Degree of synchronisation - greater synchrony increases the size of the wave

- **Behavioural state**

Excited	desynchronised with low amplitude
Alert	fast with low amplitude
Relaxed	slow with alpha bursts
Drowsy	slow with low alpha

2.1.1
Write down at least six clinical conditions in which EEG is useful and describe what abnormalities may be observed

Feedback is given over the page but try answering the question before looking

Clinical conditions:

- **Coma and altered states of awareness of uncertain aetiology**

- **Delirium**
  - typically slow wave activity, which correlates with the disturbance of consciousness (note that in delirium tremens the activity may be normal or fast)

- **Epilepsy**

  EEG showing ictal activity during a seizure is diagnostic, e.g.:
  - clonic seizure — groups of large 8 -12 Hz spikes
  - absence — 3Hz spike and wave
  - partial seizure — localised spike or sharp waves

NOTE

- *EEG record can remain normal even during an attack (e.g. Jacksonian and simple partial seizures)*
- *interictal EEG's are normal in around 30% of people with epilepsy*
- *epileptiform discharges are found in degenerative brain disorders, learning disability, psychosis and personality disorder. And rarely in normal individuals (paroxysmal bursts and excess slow activity)*

- **Head injury**
  - gauging prognosis and diagnosing post-traumatic epilepsy
  - pointing to an organic component in uncertain cases

- **Encephalitis**
  - diffuse irregular slow waves and scattered sharp waves, with slowing or reduction in alpha activity
  - seizure patterns are not uncommon in the acute stage
  - persistent slow waves indicate permanent brain damage
  - new spikes or spike and wave complexes suggests secondary epilepsy
  - subacute sclerosing panencephalitis and herpes simplex have EEG changes of high diagnostic value

- **Dementia** (differential diagnosis of pseudodementia)

  Amplitude is increased over diseased areas.
  - Alzheimer's - slowed/alpha
  - Pick's - reduced frontal activity
  - CJD - bilateral 3 Hz waves (characteristic) with startle myoclonus
  - Huntington's - flattened trace - excess theta with low voltage

- **Space occupying lesions**
  - focal delta wave focus in cerebral tumours

- **Cerebral infarctions**
  - gauging prognosis; minimal changes with early resolution predict favourable outcome and normal EEG with neurological symptoms suggests little further clinical improvement

- **Metabolic disorders**
  - sensitive indicator of cerebral insufficiency

- **Drug effects**
  - neuroleptics; increased theta and delta activity
  - tricyclics; increased theta and delta with reduced alpha
  - hypnotics; increased theta and beta (especially frontal)
  - alcohol; increased theta (becoming delta with paroxsysm on withdrawal)

2.1.2

The following recording is characterised by semi-rhythmic slow activity at the back of the head (leads 3,4,7 and 8)

Under what circumstances might this be normal?

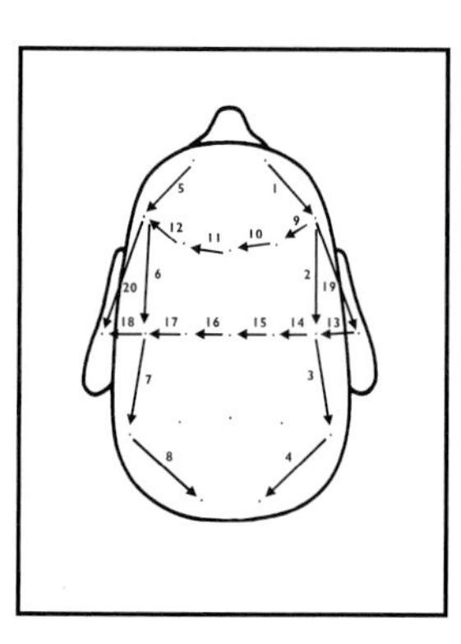

Bipolar transverse

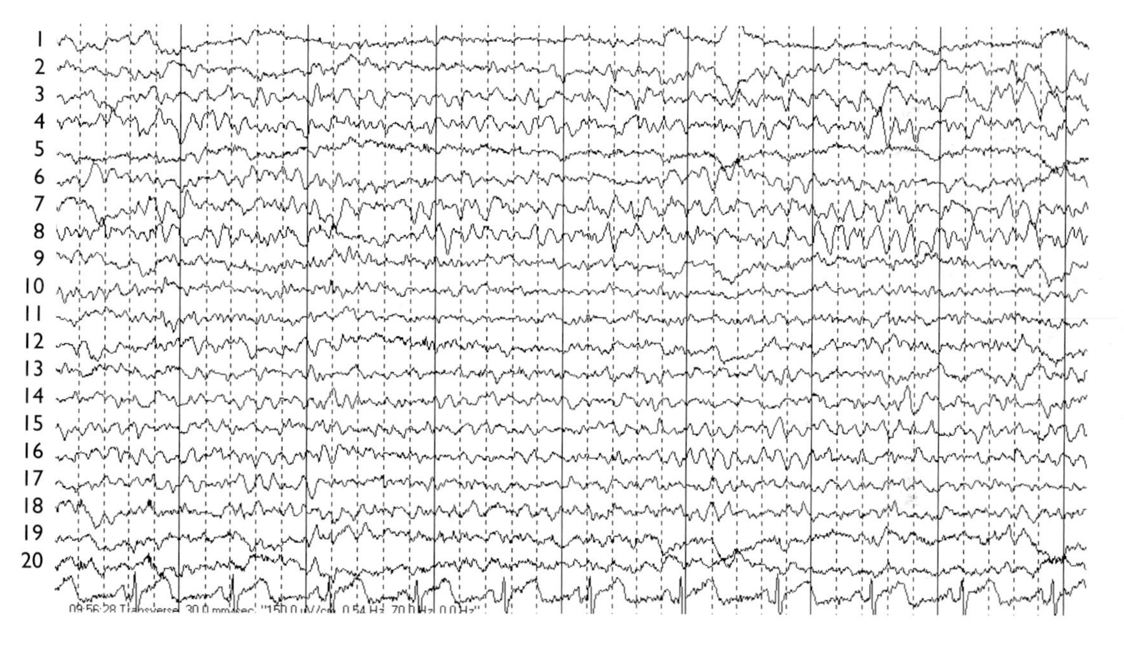

2.1.3

What state do you think the patient was in when this recording was made?

(note the spikey event in the middle of both recordings)

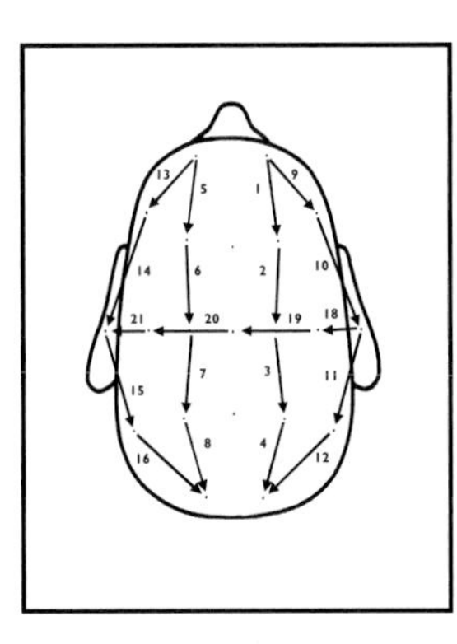

Bipolar double banana

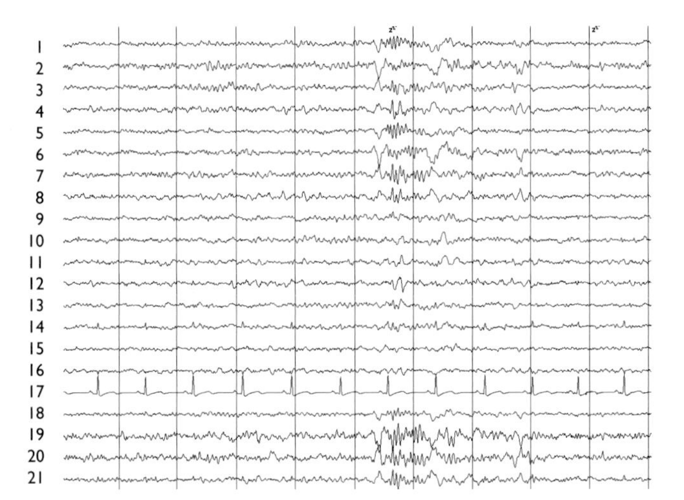

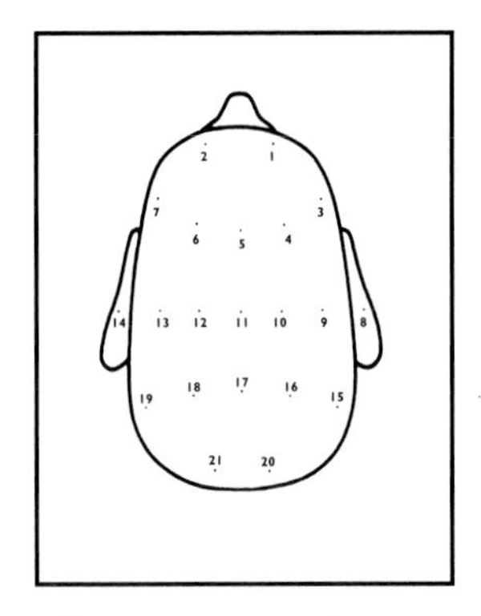

Common average reference

1
2
3
4
5
6
7
8
9
10
11
12
13
14
15
16
17
18
19
20
21

14:38:46 Average 30.0 mm/sec 70.0µV/cm 0.54 Hz 70.0 Hz 0.0 Hz

2.1.4

Effect of three minutes vigorous hyperventilation in a 28 year old.

Is this response normal?

(focus on leads 1 and 9)

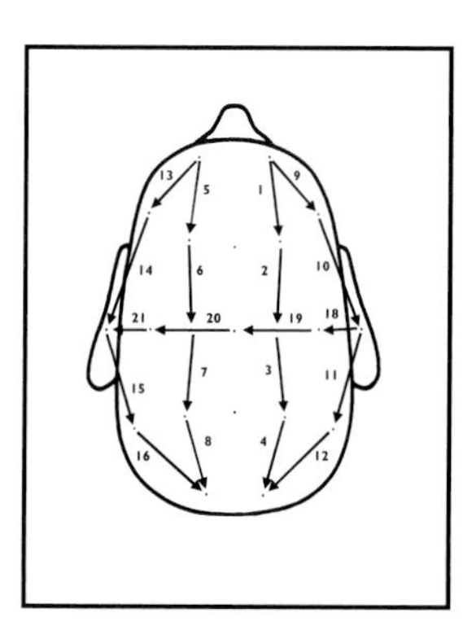

Bipolar double banana

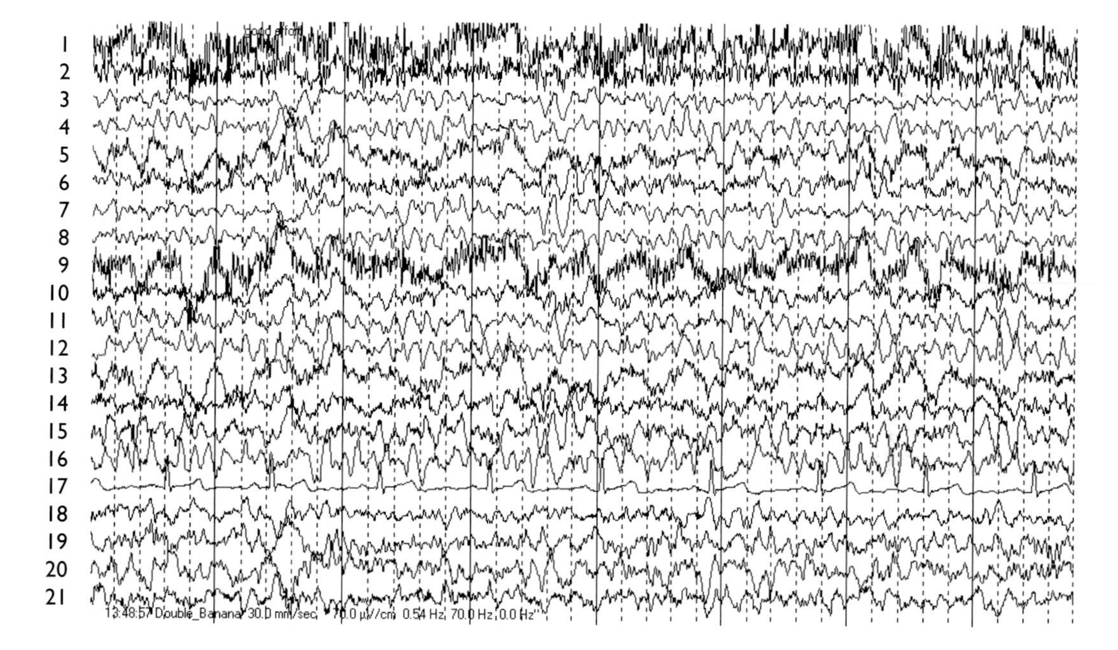

2.1.5
What is the main difference between these two EEGs?
(state what each shows)

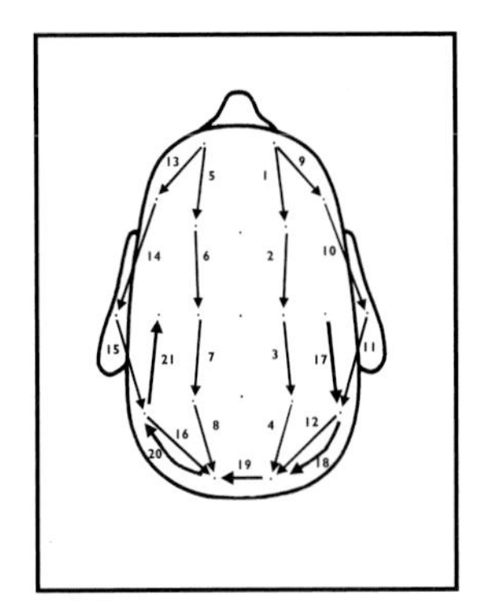
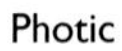
Photic

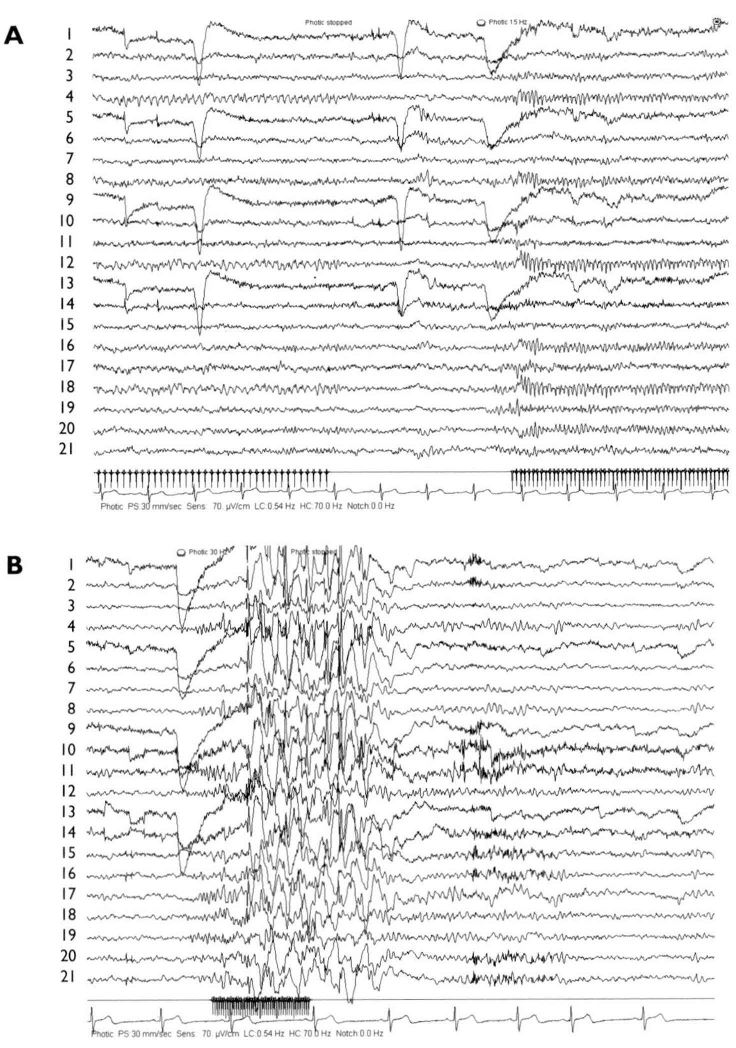

2.1.6
What does this EEG show and what is the most likely clinical comcomitant?

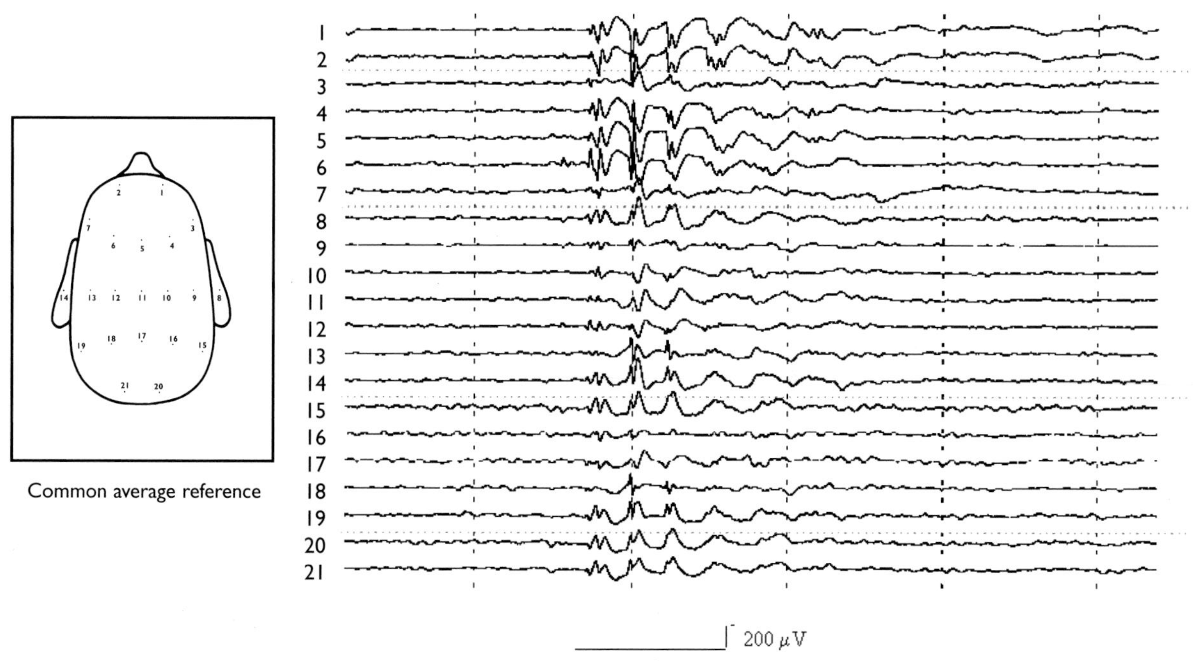

Common average reference

2.1.7
What clinical condition is identified by these two recordings?

These two EEGs are taken from the same patient, on two separate occasions

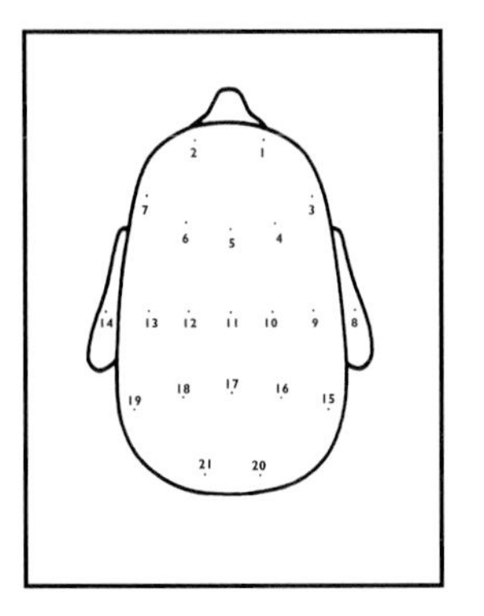

Common average reference

A

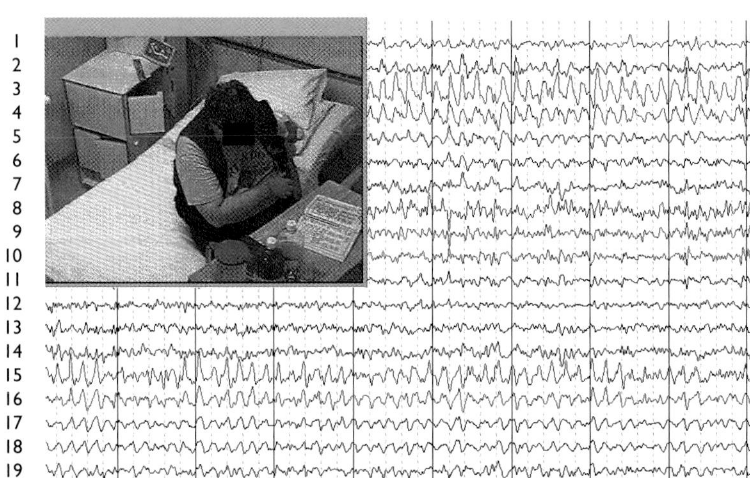

B

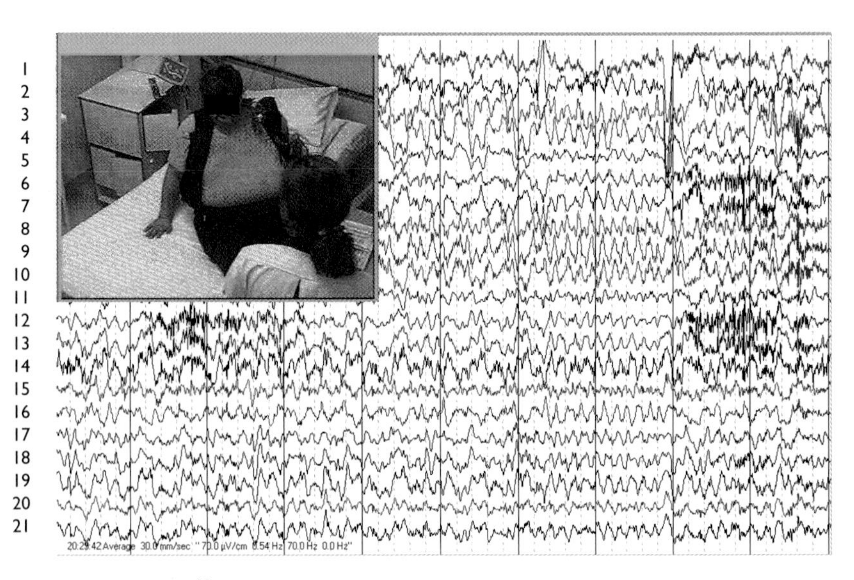

2.1.8
What abnormalities does this EEG show and which side is more abnormal?

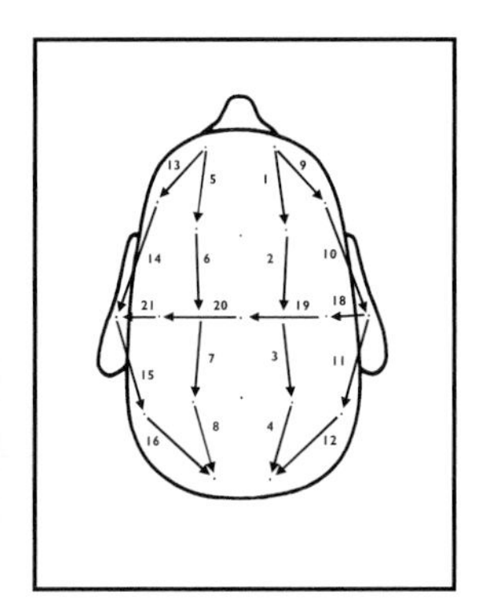

Bipolar double banana

1
2
3
4
5
6
7
8
9
10
11
12
13
14
15
16
17
18
19
20
21

16:36:41 Double_Banana 30.0 mm/sec "100.0 µV/cm 0.54 Hz 70.0 Hz 0.0 Hz"

2.1.2

- **Posterior slow waves of youth (PTSW)**

The semi-rhythmic activity (in leads 3,4,7 and 8) are delta waves, localised in the posterior temporal regions representing posterior slow waves of youth. These finally disappear early in the third decade in most subjects but can often be misinterpreted as abnormal when observed (the subject was 11 years old).

NOTE - Age changes

The infant's EEG is dominated by slow activity, an alpha rhythm appearing in the second year of life. Through childhood and adolescence much more theta and delta activities are seen than in adults - the recording is polyrhythmic. The EEG remains fairly stable through middle age, and starts to progressively change after the fifth decade - presumably as a function of cerebral degenerative and vascular pathology. In the elderly, slowing of the record and the occurrence of sharp transients over the temporal regions are common, and not necessarily of clinical significance.

2.1.3

- **Deep sleep - sleep spindles/K-complexes**

The patient is deeply asleep. In drowsiness, the alpha rhythm disappears and the record is dominated by beta and/or theta activity. With increasing depth of sleep the record slows, with delta activity preponderant in deep sleep. Various transients occur, such as; frontal bursts at 10 to 14/sec, sleep spindles, sharp waves or sharp and slow K-complexes at the vertex in relation to arousal in moderate to deep sleep, and sharp waves at the back of the head (Parieto-Occipital Sharp transients of sleep, or POSTS).

NOTE - Sleep activation

Sleep may occur spontaneously in the EEG lab or be induced following sleep deprivation or by medication. During sleep, epilepiform activity occurs more readily. Sleep activation forms an essential part of EEG investigation of epilepsy.

2.1.4

- **Hyperventilitaion - normal EEG response**

Three minutes vigorous hyperventilation slows the EEG, and in young subjects produces bifrontal delta activity (shown in leads I and 9). In a younger age group there may be more prominent rhythmic delta activity but in adults some slowing is usual. EEG abnormalities, such as focal slowing may be increased or unmasked and epileptiform activity elicited. In particular, generalised spike-and-wave activity or absence seizures are activated.

2.1.5

- **Photic stimulation: normal /abnormal**

Flicker stimulation at frequencies up to 60 flashes/sec normally elicits brain activity synchronous with the flashes (EEG 'A'). In photosensitive epilepy a generalised 'photoparoxysmal response' may be elicited (as shown by a generalised, hypersynchronous response in EEG 'B')

NOTE - Photic activation

The main role of photic activation is in epilepsy, as some 5% of epileptic patients are photosensitive and commonly suffer visually induced seizures.

2.1.6

- **Absence seizure**
  EEG shows generalised spike and wave discharge (3 Hz) occuring in an absence seizure. Note the symmetrical onset and ending, characteristic of generalised seizures.

2.1.7

- **Complex partial seizure** (occuring during telemetry)
  Although both traces are of the same patient they are distinguished by the fact that one shows a clearly lateralised right sided discharge (EEG 'A') whereas the other shows bilateral rhythmic sharp waves (EEG 'B'). Neither shows a clear focus; this is usually the case with recordings of complex partial seizures.

▸▸EEG in epilepsy pp 231-2

2.1.8

- **Dysplasia**
  EEG shows excess theta activity more prominent on the left than the right (partial epilepsy due to cortical dysplasia)

See also

▸▸ Other uses of EEG pp 131-3
- *Event related potentials (ERP)*
- *Brain electrical activity mapping (BEAM)*
- *Fractal analysis*
- *Magnetoencephalography*

2.2 - NEUROIMAGING

Neuroimaging can be subdivided into structural and functional. The next few pages contain examples of three main types of structural neuroimaging being used in these modules, namely Plain X-ray/CT/MRI. Neuroimaging is increasingly superior to all other investigations in terms of localising pathology. The aim of this section is to highlight some of the radiological findings of neuropathological conditions that you may well encounter in your clinical work and help you to be able to detect and interpret these changes. In the clinical context, indications that would support the need for a scan of your patient's brain would include; atypical presentations, rapidily progressing conditions or conditions with prominent focal neurological features.

NOTE - Standard views

When viewing a transverse or axial scan, it's conventional to have the frontal lobes at the top of the picture and the occipital lobes at the bottom. Imagine yourself looking up at the scan from underneath, making the left hemisphere appear on the right and vice versa. Other views possible with MRI include coronals (highlighting both hemispheres) and sagitals (frontal - occipital plane)

- ***Radiography of the skull pp 135-48***
  You may wish to refer to these pages as you work through this section.
- ***Neuroimaging in head injury pp 165-6, tumours pp 231, epilepsy pp 289 and dementia pp 433-4***
  This reference is given for additional reading

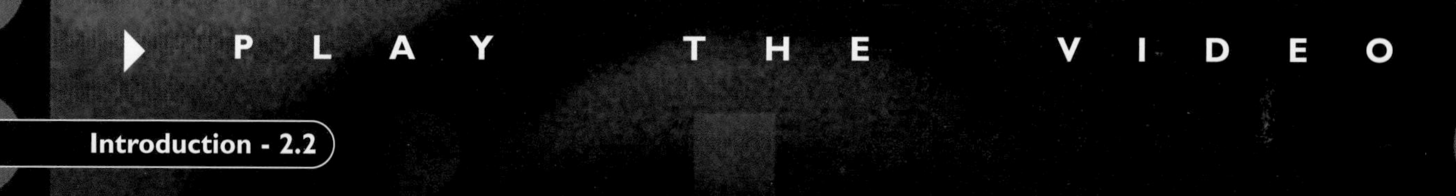

Introduction - 2.2

Excerpt 2.2 features Dr Dawson with Professor Goldberg, discussing structural neuroimaging.

Watch the video and stop when prompted. There is no exercise based on this excerpt; it's included for an introductory demonstration. When you've seen the excerpt, browse through the example over the next six pages before trying the exercise that follows.

Plain radiographs detect only four basic densities; bone (and/or calcification), air, fat and contrast medium. Detection is then only possible when one density abutts one of the other three.

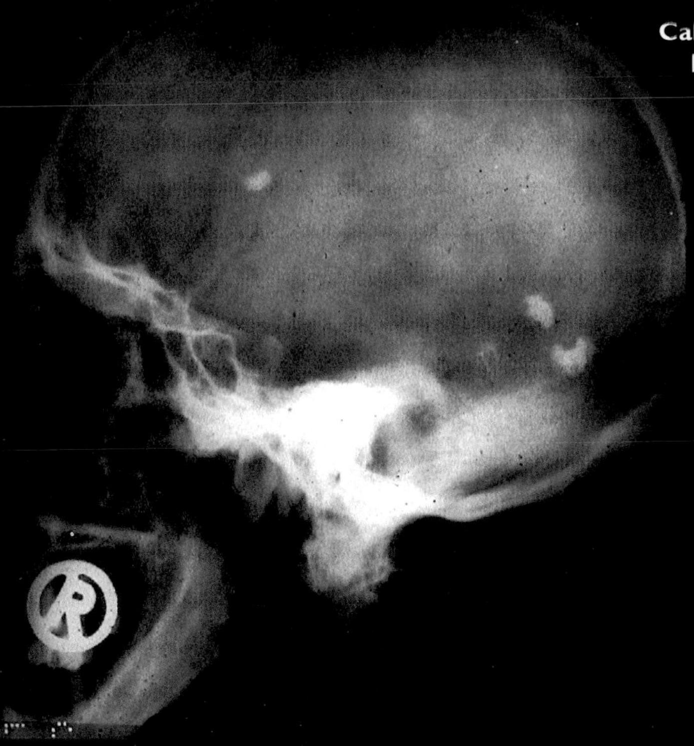

Calcification - Cysticercosis

Lateral and anteriorposterior views of the skull. The scan shows abnormally dense lesions which stand out against the normal skull bone density. These abnormalities represent remnants of calcified cysticerci.

Note that calcification occurs in other infections and certain tumours

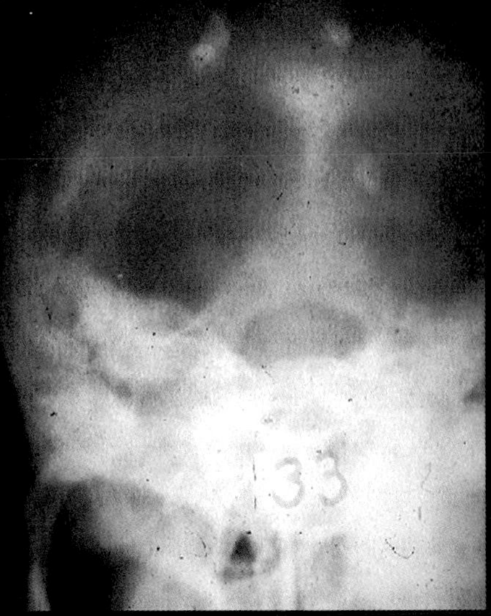

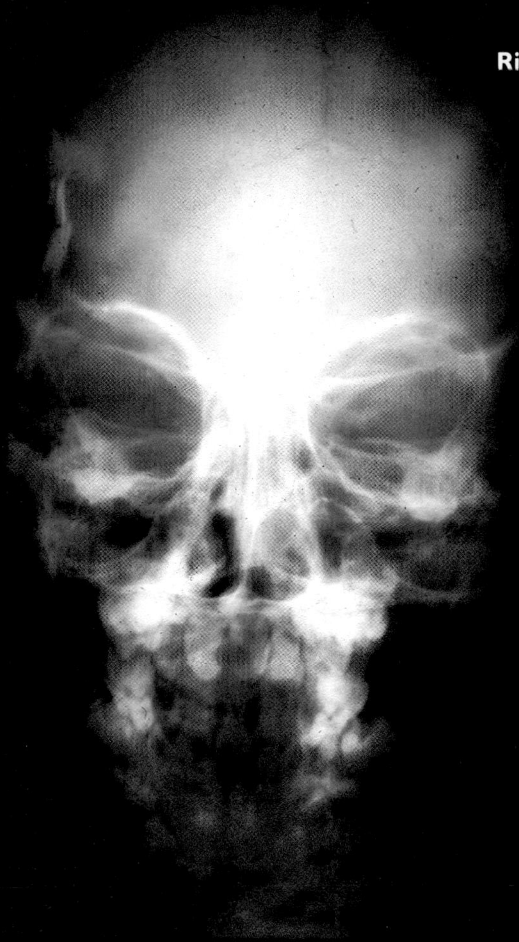

Right sided skull fracture

Anterioposterior view showing depressed fracture with buckled bony fragments.

Note the appearance of air in the sinuses and nose (absence of densities).

CT has the advantage over plain X-ray in detecting subtleties in soft tissue - ie features within the brain, for example the basal ganglia, internal capsule and grey/white matter interface.

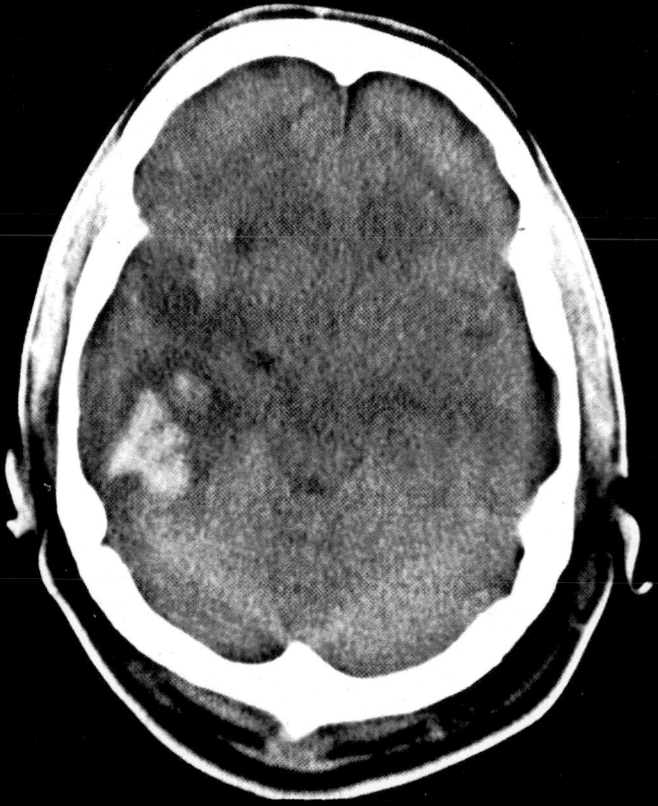

Δ Right temporal intracranial haemorrhage

This axial view shows lobulated, high attenuated large and small white lesions in the right posterior temporal lobe. Being white suggests fresh haemorrhage not just calcification. The low attenuation black surrounding is oedema and/or areas of infarction.

NOTE

You can tell it's the temporal lobe by its location in line with the ears.

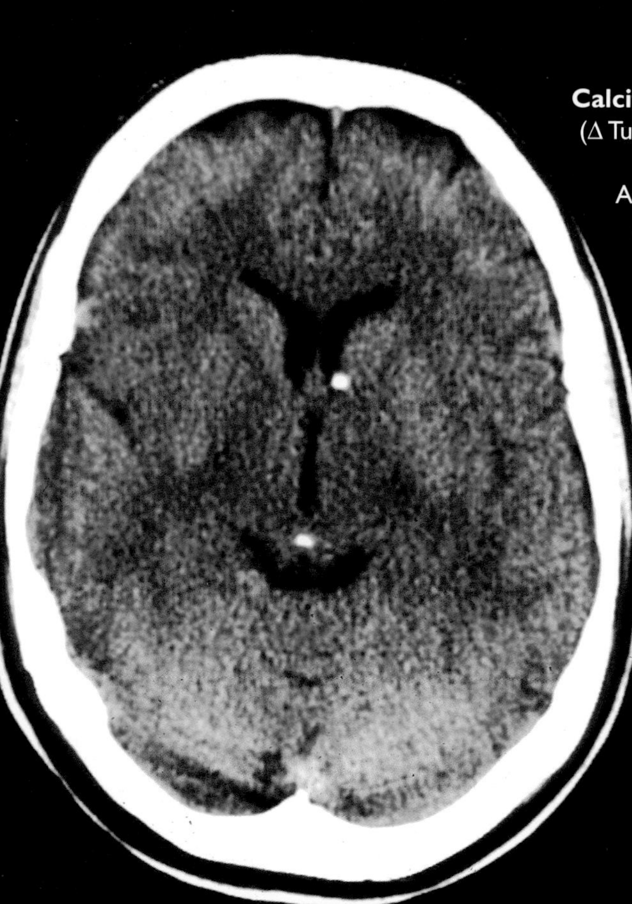

Calcification
(Δ Tuberous Sclerosis)

Axial view showing high density lesions on the surface of the left ventricle. Distinction in grey and white matter and internal capsule is clearly shown, as is the cortical grey mantle.

Jnlike CT scanning, MRI involves no X-irradiation, but makes ɹse of the magnetic properties of nuclei and their capacity to be excited by radiofrequency pulses. The fine detail of the mages produced is comparable with the macroscopic detail seen at post-mortem. It is better at detecting residua of brain njury, infections and the plaques of Multiple sclerosis. Also the posterior fossa and pituatary are more clearly visible as there s no bone artifact. Unlimited views are available using different requencies, each optimised to differentially visuslise anatomy and pathology. The two commonest sequences (T1 and 2 weighted) are shown here. A simple way to tell them apart is that the CSF is black with T1 and white with T2.

NOTE

MRI cannot be performed if there is any magnetic material present either in the body (e.g. cardiac pacemaker) or attached to the body

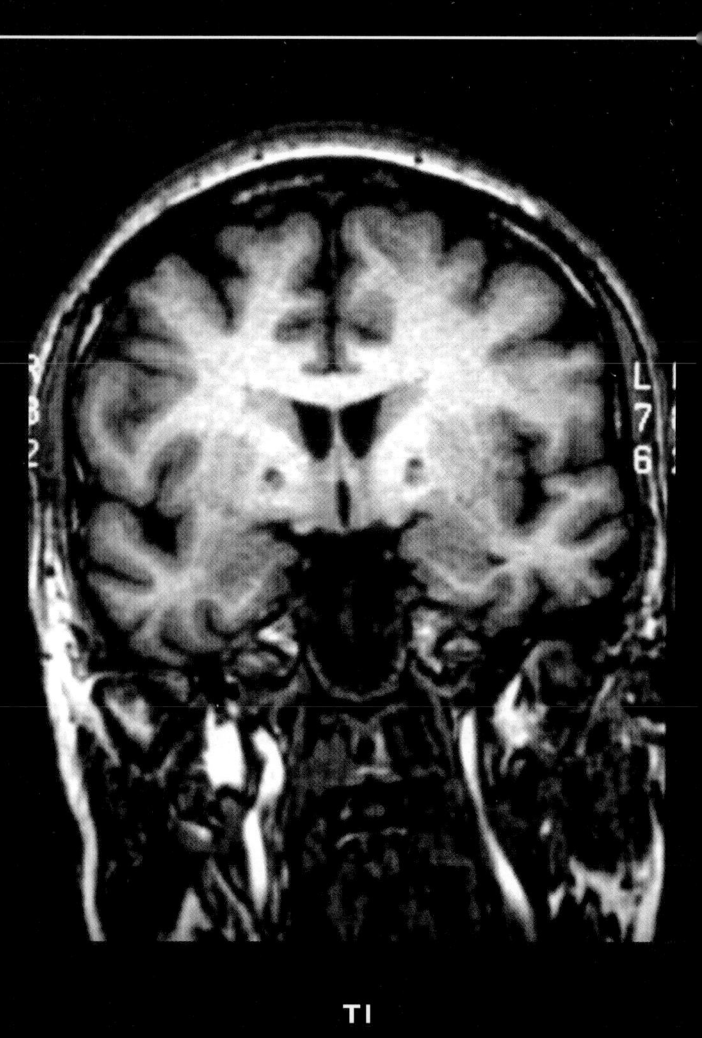

T1

Bilateral globus pallidus necrosis

(Δ carbon monoxide poisoning)

T1 - Coronal view showing black lesions bilaterally in the globus pallidus with black CSF. T1 weighted images are better at visualising normal anatomy (note the clear visualisation of

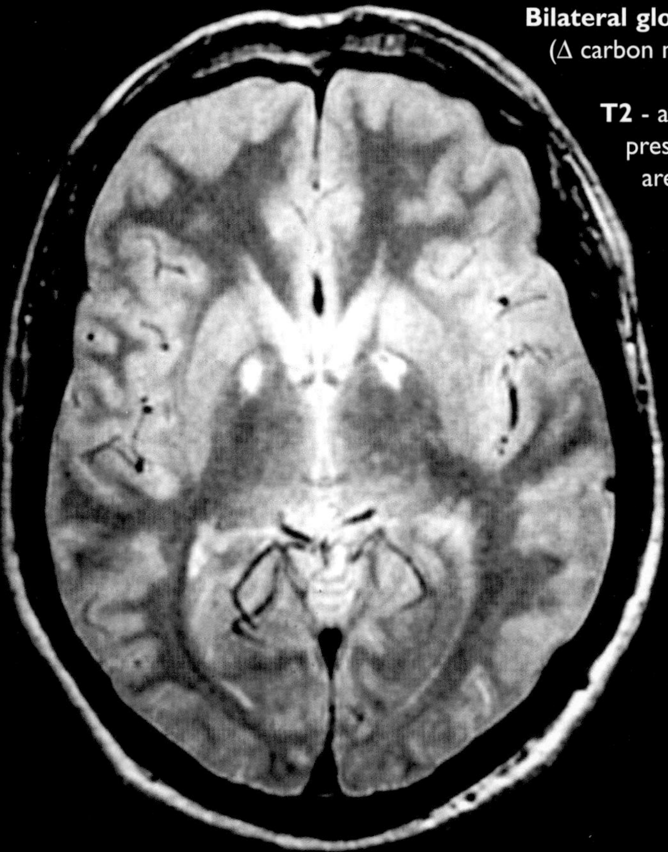

Bilateral globus pallidus necrosis (same patient)
(Δ carbon monoxide poisoning)

T2 - axial image showing bilateral high signal (white lesions) and the presence of the middle and posterior cerebral arteries. T2 views are better for visualising pathology (high white signal).

T2

Other views:

- **Proton density;** intermediate between T1 and T2 images
  - *Plate 5 pg xviii*
- **Contrast** (e.g. Gadalinium usually); often may distinguish tumours from surrounding oedema and highlights vessels

FUNCTIONAL IMAGING

Functional imaging, previously predominantly a research tool, is increasingly clinically useful when facilities are available.

- **Functional MRI (fMRI)**
  Image generated from minute changes in regional blood flow and/or oxygenation in relation to local physiological activity, providing a high resolution brain map of areas involved in discrete tasks and activities.

  ›› *Functional MRI pp 143-4*
  ›› *Plate 4 e.g. schizophrenia pg xviii*
  ›› *Plate 6 e.g. 3D surface rendering of MRI images*

- **Positron Emission Tomography (PET)**
  Cross-sectional image of brain radioactivity, highlighted by an injected labelled radioisotope, yielding information on the site and rate of dynamic processes such as metabolism and cerebral blood flow (often in areas not otherwise accessible). A cyclotron is required to generate the short-lived isotopes and complex data analysis is required to make the task state/control state subtractions. An example of it's clinical usefulness is when a small lesion on MRI is shown to be a large functional deficit on PET.

  ›› *Positron emission tomography pp 144-7*
  ›› *Plate 1 and 2 15O-PET in phonological task pg xvii*
  ›› *Plate 3 133Xe-PET in schizophrenia and normal control pg xvii*

- **Single Photon Emission Computerised Tomography (SPECT)**
  This procedure is used to determine the 3D distribution of radiopharmacological agents. It is an elaboration of radioisotope scanning, and although less sensitive than PET, yields high quality images. Examples of the clinical usefulness of SPECT include:
  - **Stroke** - decreased frontal uptake
  - **Alzheimer's** - decreased uptake in tempropariental regions
  - **Multi-infarct dementia** - focal deficits
  - **Huntington's** - decreased uptake in the head of the caudate

  ›› *Single photon emission computerised tomography pp147-8*
  ›› *Plate 7 normal subject pg xix*

Exercise 2.2

The scans featuring in this next series cover a range of radiological manifestations of cerebral pathology. Study each scan carefully; then write down an answer to the following question:

What abnormal features do you think are present and what condition(s) could possibly lead to these features?
Answers are given at the end of the exercise, but try writing an answer to each example before turning to look

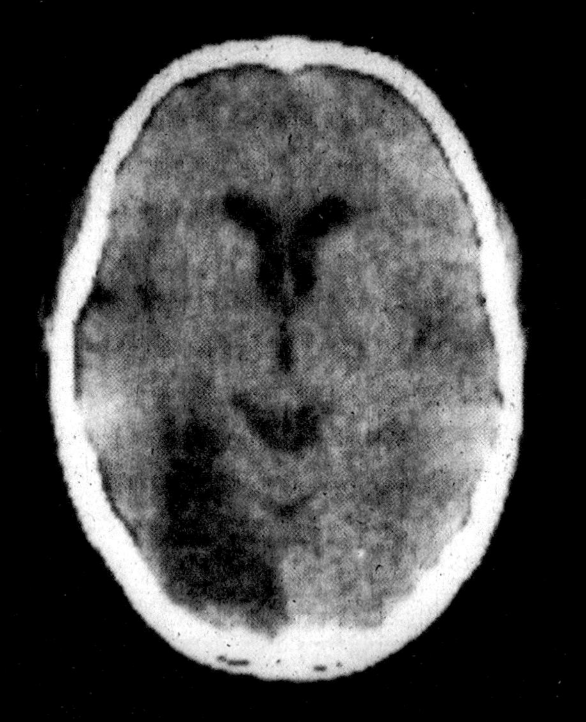

2.2.1

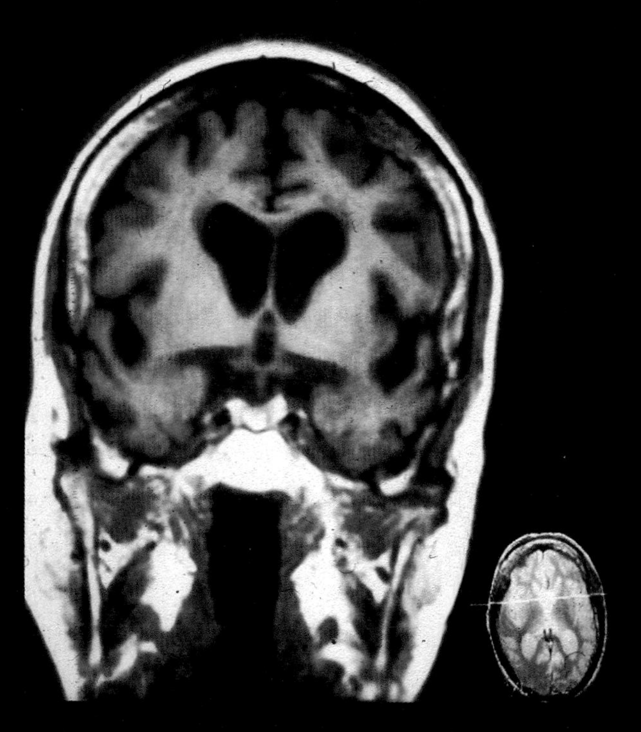

2.2.2

2.2.3

2.2.4

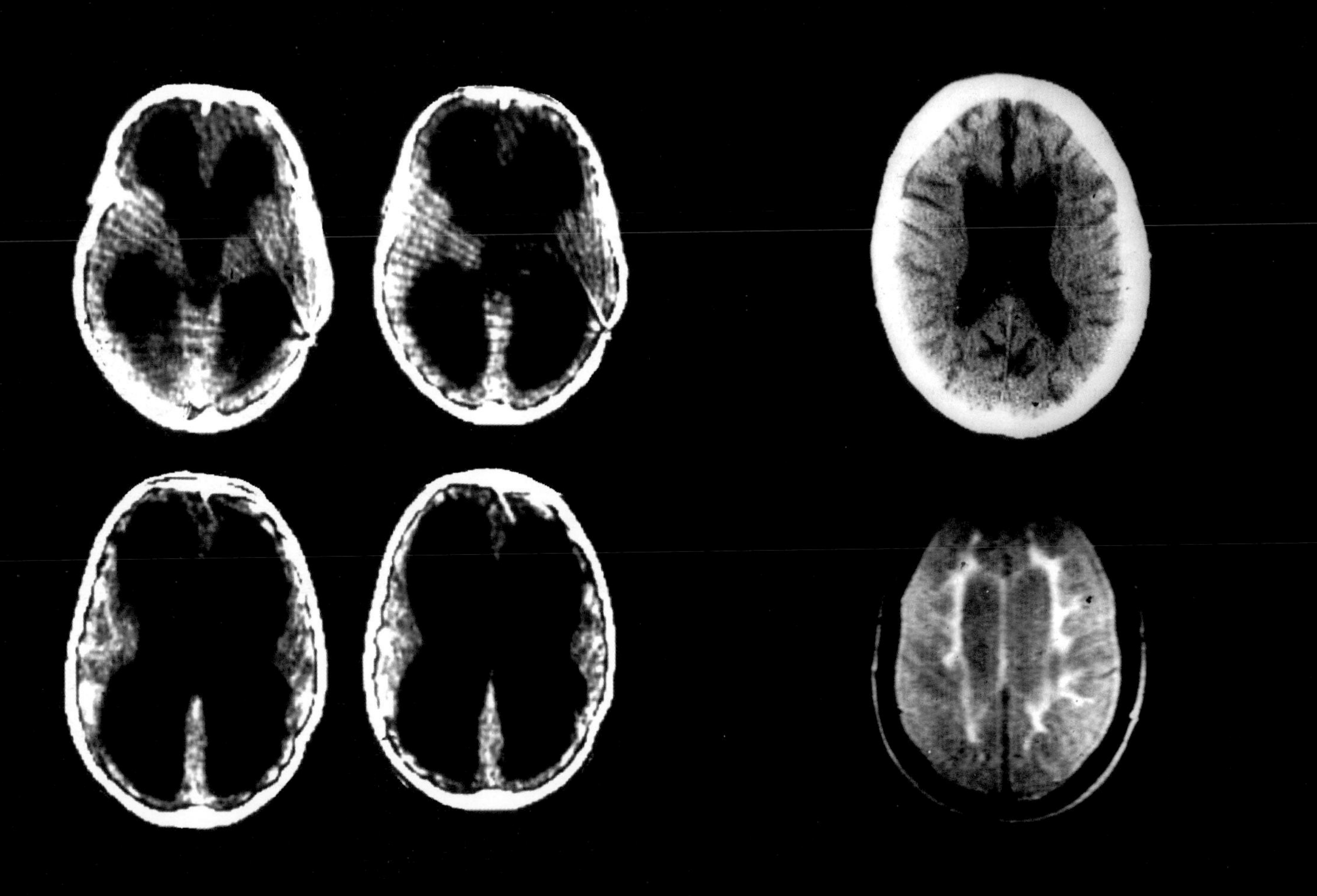

2.2.5

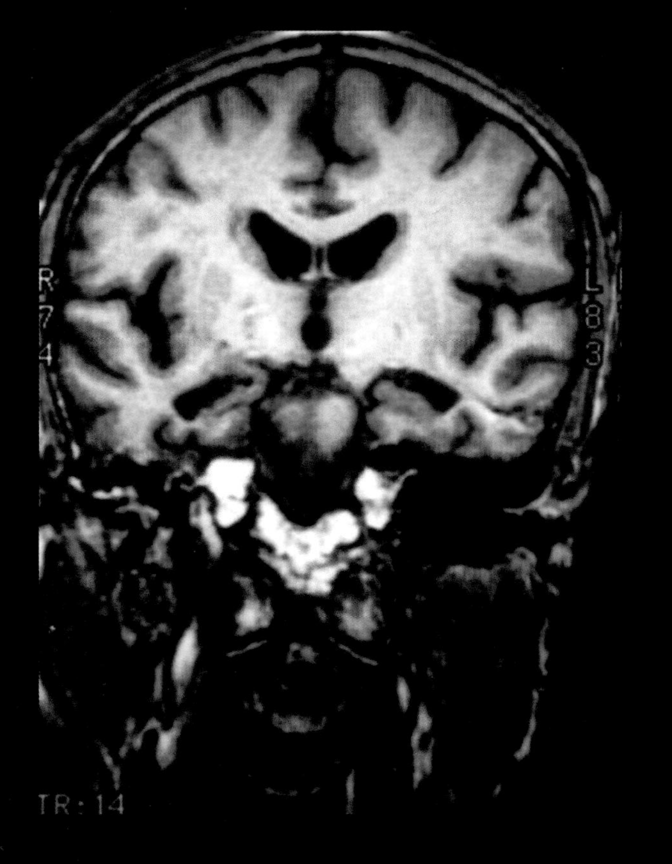

2.2.6

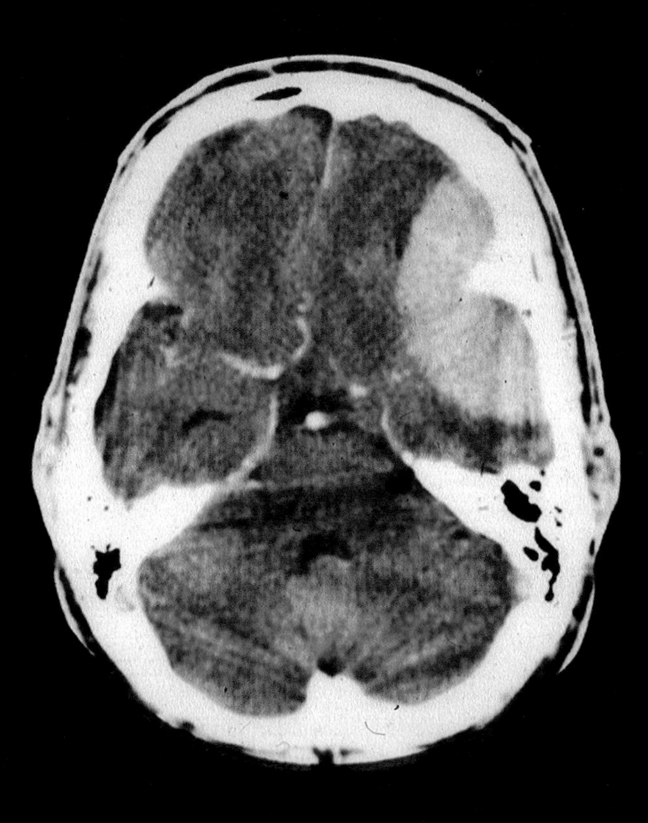

2.2.1

- **Axial CT - black lesion in right tempro-occipital region**
  The two white areas adjacent to the brain edge are, in this case, bony artifacts.
- **Infarction involving the optic radiation and visual cortex** (ΔΔ tumour)
  This is an example of non-haemorrhaging lesion for which aspirin could be prescribed. A haemorrhaging lesion, for which you wouldn't prescribe aspirin, would appear white.
  (This scan is taken from the case of word blindness in module 1)

    ▸▸ ***Cerebrovascular accidents pp 375-92***

2.2.2

- **MRI (T1) coronal - preferential atrophy**
  Widening of the choroidal fissure and insula (sylvian fissure), against a background of generalised atrophy.
- **Alzheimer's disease**

    ▸▸ ***Significance of cerebral atrophy pp 138-41***

2.2.3

- **CT axial slices - gross lateral ventricle dilitation**
  Virtually no cerebral tissue is seen above the level of the brain stem and third ventricle
- **Obstructive Hydrocephalus**
  The scan comes from a 15 year old girl who was referred for anxiety and topographical diorientation.

    ▸▸ ***Hydrocephalus pp 744-50***

2.2.4

- **CT - signs of early cortical atrophy** (mild widening of sulci and ventricular enlargement)
- **MRI (T2) - focal white matter abnormalities (high white signals) affecting the ventricular surfaces**
- **Metachromatic leucodystrophy**
  (ΔΔ ischaemic vascular disease and normal ageing)
  Abnormality of neurolipid metabolism leading to dementia or motion disorder. Psychotic signs may manifest first, being replaced by widespread cognitive dysfunction later. The condition is commonly misdiagnosed as schizophrenia, presenile dementia or MS on clinical grounds.

    ▸▸ ***Metachromatic leucodystrophy pp 758-9***

2.2.5

- **MRI coronal (T1): bilateral Hippocampal atrophy**
  Wide temporal horns and flat hippocampae especially on the right
- **Hypoglycaemic coma**

    ▸▸ ***Hypoglycaemia pp 539-46***

2.2.6

- **CT scan (following contrast) - Left skull hyperostosis**
  White triangular lesion) with mushroom-like calcified mass (less dense)
- **Meningioma**
  (ΔΔ frontotemporal dementia and sarcoid)

    ▸▸ ***Tumours pp 218-36***
    ▸▸ ***Sarcoidosis pp763-5***

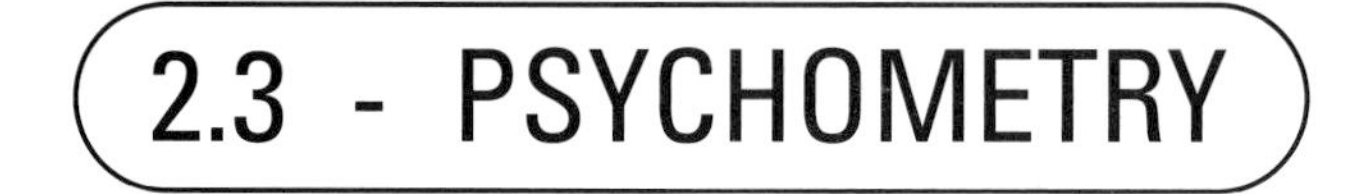

2.3 - PSYCHOMETRY

Collaboration with a clinical psychologist can aid in diagnosis and management, helping to identify dysfunction and areas of preserved function. Psychometric tests are useful in several ways; providing 'norms' against which individual variation can be measured, giving an indication as to whether brain damage or other factors are contributing to the persons profile of cognitive impairment, and providing a baseline to track changes and chart progress.

Psychometric tests can broadly be subdivided into those measuring a number of different areas of cognitive functioning. For each cognitive domain, specific tests as well as test batteries are often available. Although some of them are listed over the page (and further discussed in 'Organic Psychiatry'), each clinical psychologist may have their own preferences for the combination of tests used, especially given the rapidly increasing number of new tests available.

Psychometric tests are constantly being re-developed. Often a test developed and validated in one country won't export to another country due to cultural differences

⏩ ***Psychometric assessment pp 108-22***
Details of the tests used are covered in these pages. You may wish to use them as reference during this section.

▶ PLAY THE VIDEO

Introduction 2.3

Excerpt 2.3 features Dr Goldstein with Dr Church, discussing some general issues relating to psychometry.

Watch the video and stop when prompted. This is an introductory piece; no questions are being asked. Familarise yourself with the tests listed overleaf before tackling the two vignettes that make up the exercises in this section.

PSYCHOMETRIC TESTS

NOTE

Some test batteries, such as the Halstead-Reitan Battery, measure a number of the functions below and you would need to use other cognitive tests (e.g. the WAIS, WAIS-R) to supplement the information it yields.

INTELLIGENCE

Battery of tests:

- **Wechsler Adult Intelligence Scale** (WAIS, WAIS-R, WAIS-III)

Specific tests:

- **Raven's Progressive Matrices** (Advanced, Standard, Coloured)
- **National Adult Reading Test (NART)** (to assess pre-morbid IQ)

PERCEPTION

Battery of tests:

- **Visual Object and Space Perception Battery**
- **Behavioural Inattention Test**

Specific tests:

- **Bender-Gestalt Test**
- **Benton Line Orientation Test** *(not described in your textbook but widely used)*

LANGUAGE

Battery of tests:

- **Speed and Capacity of Language Processing**

Specific tests:

- **Boston Naming Test**
- **Graded Naming Test**
- **Token Test**

MEMORY

Battery of tests:

- **Wechsler Memory Scale** (WMS, WMS-R, WMS-III)
- **Adult Memory and Information Processing Battery**
- **Rivermead Behavioural Memory Test**

Category of test (measuring a particular memory function):

- **Paired Associate Learning Tests**
- **List Learning Tests**

Specific tests:

- **Recognition Memory Tests**
- **Benton Visual Retention Test**
- **Rey-Osterrieth Test**
- **Synonym Learning Test**
- **Kendrick Object Learning Test**

FRONTAL LOBE (EXECUTIVE FUNCTION)

Battery of tests:

- **Behavioural Assessment of Dysexecutive Syndrome** (includes Strategy Application Tests)

Category of test (measuring a particular executive function):

- **Verbal Fluency Tests** (letter based, semantic categories)
- **Design fluency**

Specific tests:

- **Wisconsin Card Sorting Test**
- **Stroop Tests**
- **Cognitive Estimates Test**
- **Trail Making Test**

VIGILANCE

- **Paced Auditory Serial Additive Test (PASAT)**
- **Continuous Performance Test**

Exercise 2.3

This exercise covers case vignettes which highlights the usefulness of psychometric tests in two specific disorders.

VIGNETTE

Investigating a case of epilepsy

Mr J, a 40 year old man, developed regular epileptic seizures at the age of 5 years following a febrile convulsion at the age of 19 months. His schooling was not particularly disrupted by his epilepsy but he has had difficulty remaining employed because of his current seizure frequency. He is now experiencing frequent seizures despite anti-convulsant medication. He is ambidextrous. A recent MRI scan revealed right mesial temporal lobe sclerosis.

Cognitive testing with the WAIS-R revealed a Verbal I.Q. of 97 and a Performance I.Q. of 84. He did particularly poorly on the Picture Completion, Block Design and Object Assembly subtests. Performance on tests of memory and learning for verbal material fell between the 10th - 25th percentile whereas scores on analogous tests of visuospatial material fell below the 10th percentile.

2.3.1
Are his I.Q. and memory results consistent with the presence of right mesial temporal sclerosis?

2.3.2
What other possible explanations are there for his Verbal/Performance discrepancy on the WAIS-R?

2.3.3
What special factors might complicate interpretation of test results in this case?

▸▸ ***Intelligence tests pp110-11***
You may wish to refer to these pages during this vignette

2.3.1

- **I.Q. and memory results ARE consistent with right mesial temporal sclerosis**

  The significant Verbal-Performance IQ discrepancy reflects visuo-spatial difficulties. This, taken together with his poor scores on Picture Completion, Block Design and Object Assembly sub-tests, adds support for the lesion residing in the right hemisphere. He shows relatively poorer performance on the tests of learning and recall for visuospatial material which would be consistent with a right mesial temporal lobe lesion.

2.3.2

His Verbal-Performance IQ discrepancy could be affected by other factors:

- **Sedating effects of medication**
  - all Performance IQ subtests are timed whereas only one Verbal IQ subtest is timed
- **Visual difficulties**
  - detailed analysis of visual stimuli is required in the Performance IQ sub-tests
- **Motor impairment**
  - all but one of the Performance IQ subtests require good motor dexterity
- **Inter-ictal epileptiform discharges**
  - could interrupt information processing and affect performance on timed tests

2.3.3

- **Atypical cerebral representation due to ambi-dexterity**

  He is ambidextrous, and it is therefore possible that he has atypical cerebral representation of cognitive functions, especially given the early onset of his seizures. When someone is right-handed and left hemisphere dominant for language, verbal memory functions are predominantly mediated by the left hemisphere and visuo-spatial memory functions by the right hemisphere.

Investigating a case of head injury

Mr. C is a 25 year old right handed man with limited education who sustained a severe head injury when a steel ladder fell on his head from some scaffolding. He sustained a left fronto-parietal fracture with a left frontal haemorrhagic contusion and he required surgical elevation of the skull fracture and removal of the contused brain region. He was unconscious for a week, dysphasic on regaining consciousness and has been left with a residual dysarthria and a right sided hemiparesis and has had to learn to use his left hand for writing, drawing etc.

On neuropsychological assessment six months after his injury, his Verbal IQ was 78 and his Performance IQ was 71. Premorbidly he was thought to have functioned in the low average range. Current memory testing revealed learning, recall and recognition of verbal material below the 5th percentile and learning, recall and recognition of visuospatial material between the 10th-25th percentile. Object naming was in line with premorbid estimates of functioning but he was impaired on a reading test (NART) and his verbal fluency (FAS Test) and language comprehension (modified Token Test) scores were indicative of acquired impairment despite having no comprehension difficulties during normal conversation. He was significantly impaired on the Stroop Test, the Wisconsin Card Sorting Test and the Trail Making Test but not on strategy application tests.

2.3.4
Which results are fully consistent with left frontal damage?

2.3.5
What is unexpected about the WAIS-R results and how might this be explained?

2.3.6
Are the normal strategy application test results inconsistent with other test results?

2.3.7
Can his reading ability be used to assess premorbid IQ?

▸▸ ***pp 110-12 and Frontal lobe tests pp 118-20***
You may wish to refer to these pages during this vignette

2.3.4

Left frontal damage suggested by:

- **Impaired verbal fluency, impaired performance on the Stroop Test, Trail Making Test and Wisconsin Card Sorting Test.**

2.3.5

The unexpected finding is that:

- **Despite the left hemisphere injury his Verbal IQ is (non-significantly) higher than his Performance IQ.** This could be explained by the fact that his right hemiparesis has resulted in him having to learn to use his left hand, and he is thus slower at motor tasks than he would have been had he still been able to use both hands.

2.3.6

- **Normal strategy application test results ARE NOT inconsistent**
  Impairment on one measure or executive function does not necessarily predict impairment on all other measures. The range of functions mediated by the frontal lobes are assessed by different tests. Poor performance on verbal fluency tests, the Stroop, Trails and Wisconsin Card Sorting Test suggest impairments in intrinsic generation of material, response inhibition, and selective and divided attention; whereas the strategy application tests measure planning, sequencing and rule following.

2.3.7

- **His reading ability CAN'T be used to assess premorbid IQ**
  His reading ability is currently impaired as a consequence of his brain injury. Although reading ability does correlate highly with intellectual level, and reading is generally an over-learned skill which is resilient to the effects of different types of brain damage, once reading has been affected by brain damage it cannot be used to estimate premorbid functioning. When this happens educational, occupational and other demographic information has to be used to estimate premorbid IQ. In addition to the fact that his reading itself is now impaired, his residual dysarthria may make scoring a reading test unreliable and may also therefore affect the validity of using a reading score to estimate premorbid IQ.

M2 SUMMARY

We have reached the end of Module 2 which set out to give you a brief introduction of three key specialist investigations. Don't worry if some of the technical details of the investigative procedures seem hard to grasp; the important thing is that you have a familiarity with them and have the basics with which to interpret the results you obtain. Further examples of these tests will feature in the exercises acommpanying the remaining modules on specific disorders.

Simon Fleminger

Brain injury

CONTENT

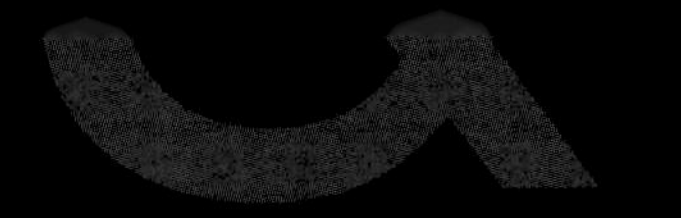

present a range of clinical conditions encountered in the brain injured patient
stress the multifactorial aetiology of psychiatric disorders following brain injury
highlight key themes of importance to a psychiatrist

objectives

By the end of this module you should be able to:

- understand the neuropathology of head injury and investigations to identify sites and types of brain damage
- know the measures of assessing the prognosis post head injury using criteria of severity
- become familarised with the acute and chronic neuropsychiatric sequelae and their management

PLAY THE VIDEO

Introduction 3.0

Excerpt 3.0 features Dr Fleminger with Professor Goldberg, discussing the assessment of brain damage and psychological factors governing the clinical picture. The need for an informant's account is emphasised.

Introduction pg 161 and Pathology and pathophysiology pp 161-6
You may wish to read the introductory paragraphs to chapter 5 and details on neuropathology before starting section 3.1

3.1 - NEUROPATHOLOGY

It's important for a psychiatrist to have an understanding of what happens to the brain in order to understand the later neuropsychiatric sequelae. The neuropathology of head injury can be arbitrarily divided into immediate (acute) and late (chronic) effects.

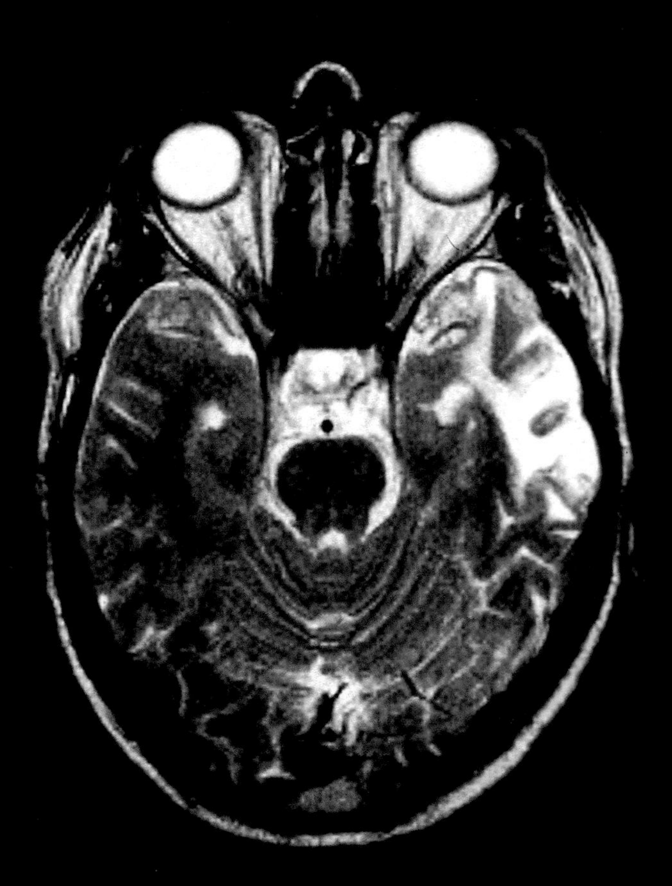

Exercise 3.1

This exercise presents a series of scans, with questions (3.1.1 - 3.1.5) to test your ability to interpret and link neuroradiological findings with brief clinical material.

Write an answer to each question before turning to the feedback.

3.1.1

This scan - an MRI (axial), T2 weighted image - was taken three months after a severe, closed head injury. The patient was unconscious for two hours. After regaining consciousness, he presented with right-sided clumsiness, memory impairment (especially verbal), slow speech and general psychomotor slowing

What neuropathology is identified and are these scan findings typical for such a condition?

3.1.2

Which of these patients is more likely to get epilepsy and why?

(Note one crucial distinction between these scans)

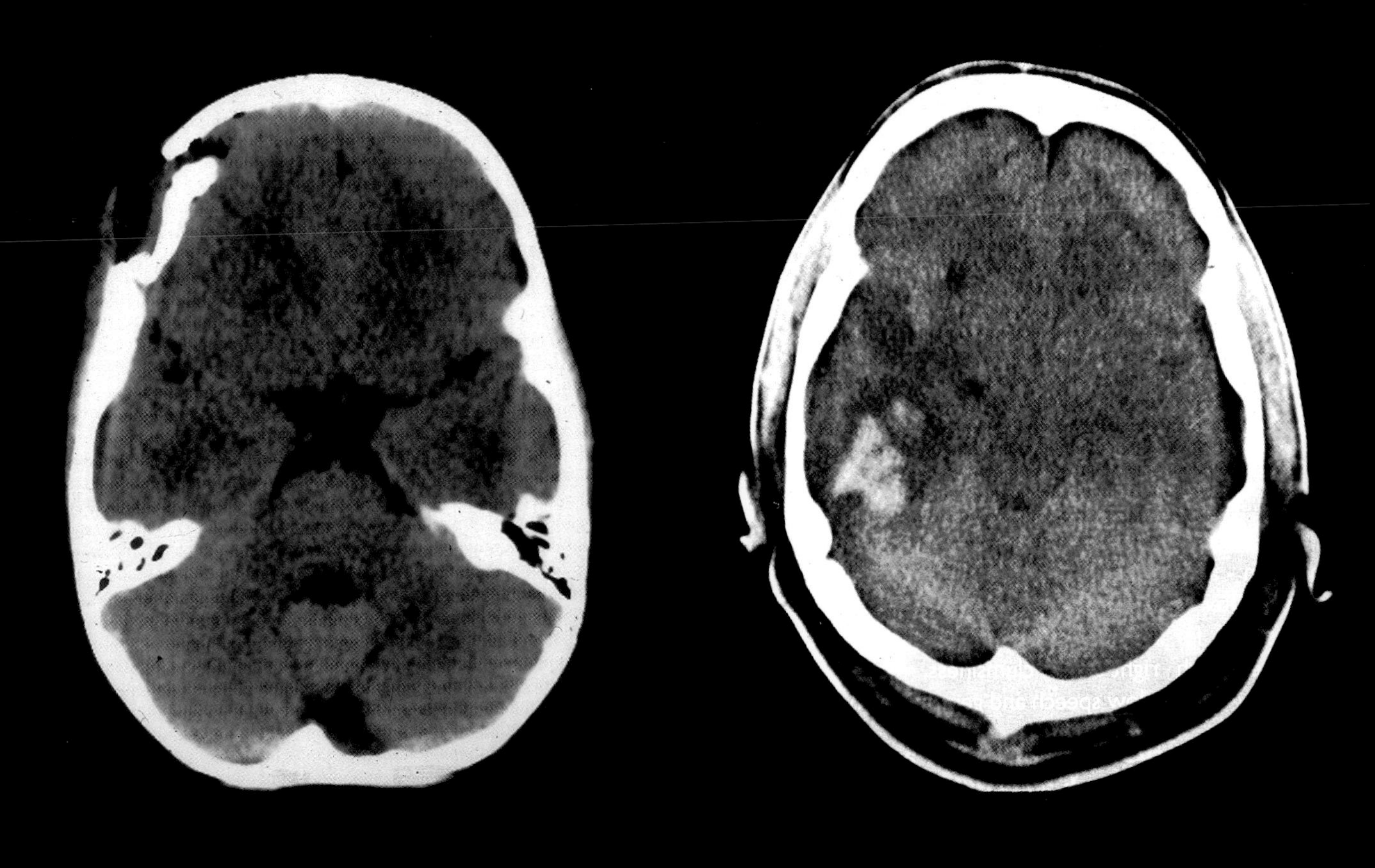

A B

3.1.3

A person trips, falls to the ground and loses consciousness for a minute. Sometime later they present with symptoms of increasing fatigue, dificulties concentrating and sleeping excessively throughout the day

Which of these two scans is more likely to have been theirs?

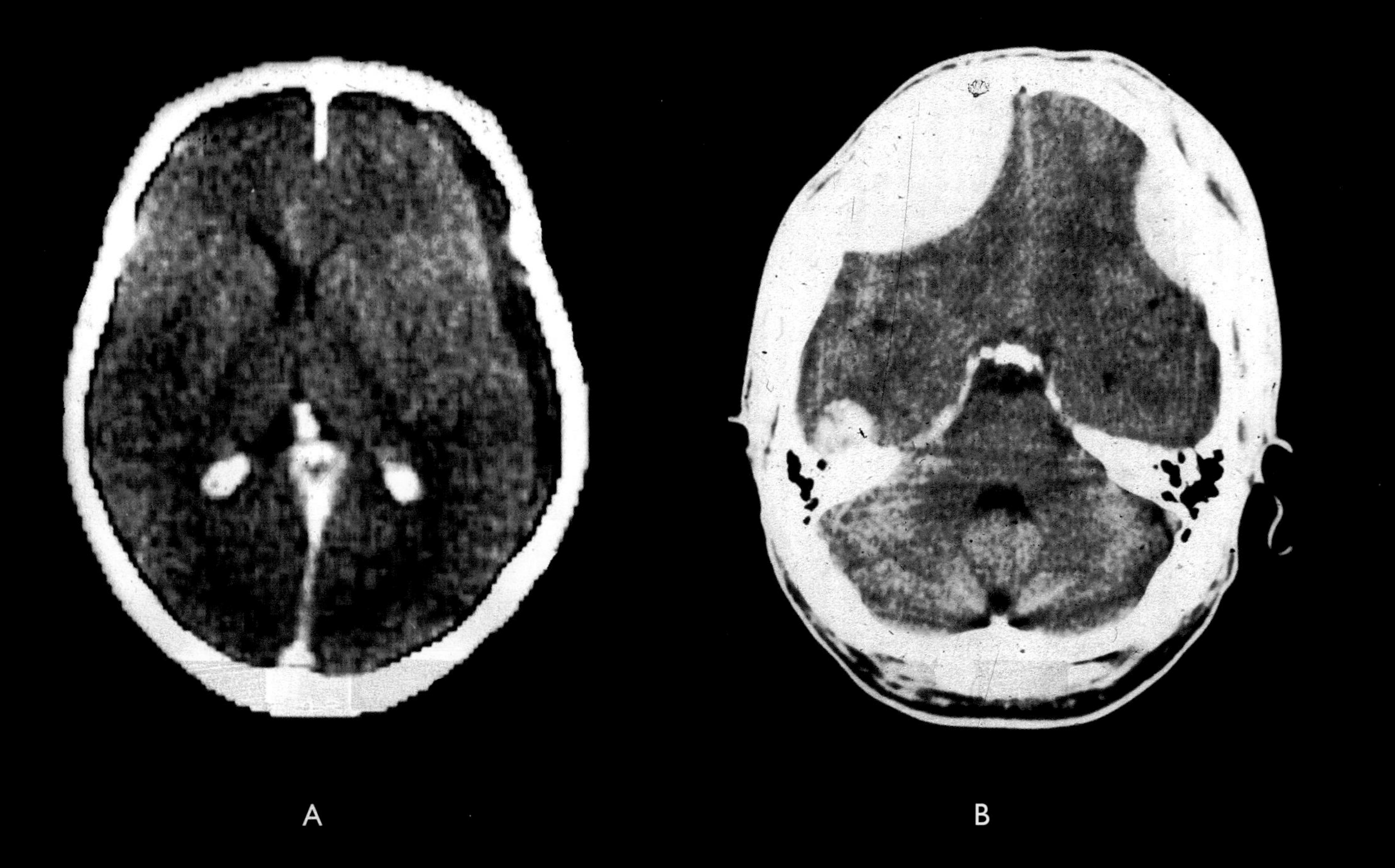

3.1.4

A patient presents with the following MRI scan. It's an axial view with proton density.

What's the neuropathology and what are the characteristic findings in someone with this condition?

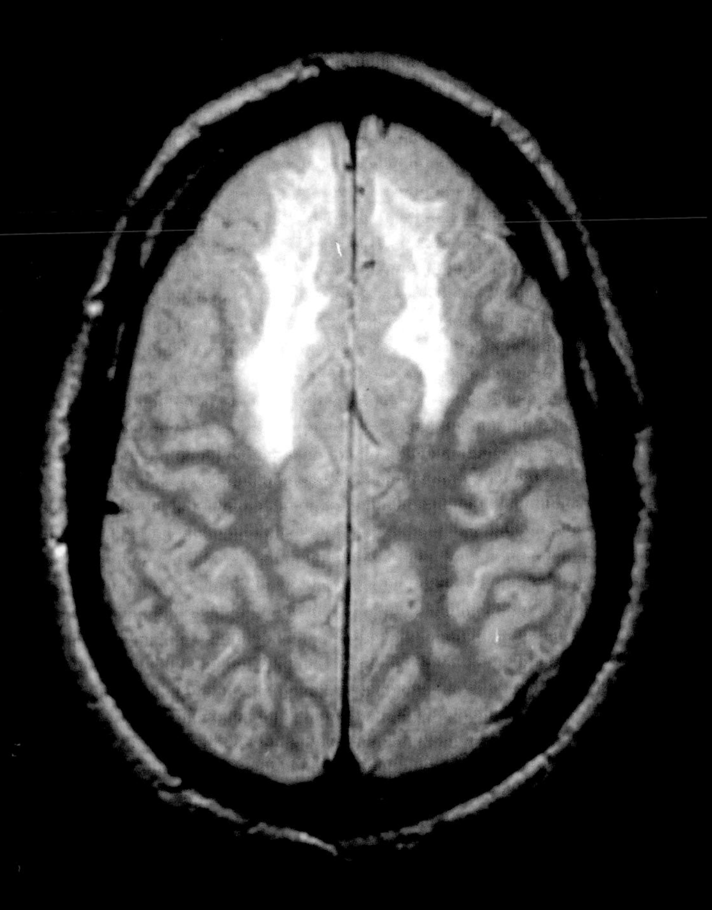

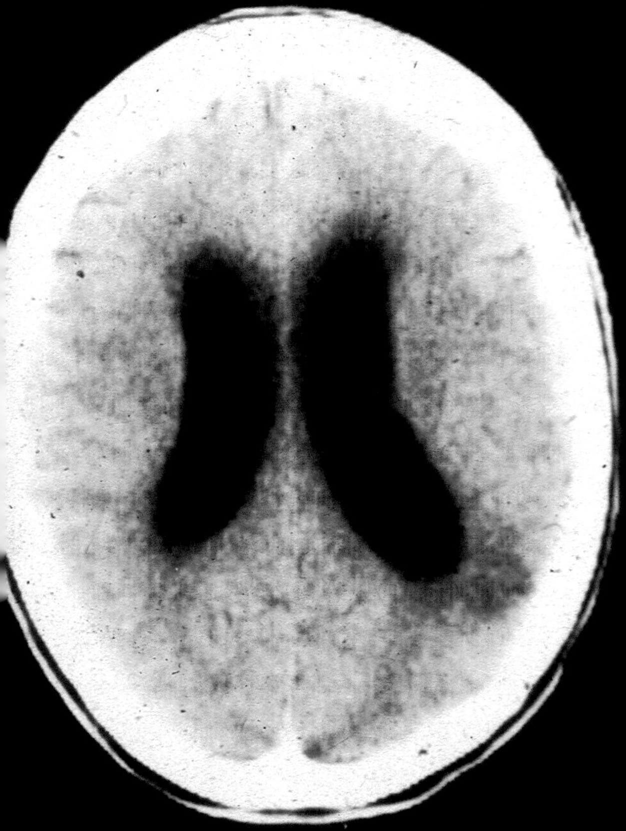

3.1.5

This is a CT scan of a patient 14 months after a very severe head injury. Two different processes could produce this picture following a closed head injury. You're informed that the brain scan of the same patient taken 4 months after the head injury was normal

What does the scan show and what processes are likely to have caused these abnormalities?

FEEDBACK

3.1.1

- **Left temporal pole contusion**
  (ΔΔ Infarction)
  The scan shows a contusion (white on T2) occupying the bulk of the left temporal pole. The findings are typical; contusions occur typically after closed head injury, where the acceleration/deceleration forces and shearing forces lead to damage from localised small vessel bleeding or local destruction. Scattered intracerebral haemorrhages are also found at the interface between grey and white matter. The location of the contusion, in the anterior temporal lobe, is typical. Medial orbital frontal surfaces is the other key area that is vulnerable to contusions. These areas correspond to sites where the brain may be traumatised against bone
  (▸▸ pg 163, column 1 for discussion)

3.1.2

- **Open head injury** (scan 'A')
  Scan 'A' is a CT image, showing a comminuted depressed fracture of the skull over the right frontal convexity. The fact that there has been a break in the skull and dural coverings would mean this qualifies as an open head injury. Open head injury is 3-5 times more likely to result in epilepsy compared with closed head injury

  Scan 'B' is a right temporal haemorrhage resulting from an internal blood vessel, and gets to be termed a closed head injury.

  ▸▸ ***Post-traumatic epilepsy pp 244-5***

3.1.3

- **Subdural haematoma** (Scan 'A')

  NOTE
  Subdurals appear concave and extradurals convex

  Scan 'A' is a CT scan showing an extensive rim of low attenuation over virtually the whole left hemisphere indicating a subdural collection of blood (probably old). Also shown is a midline shift with compression of the left lateral ventricle frontal horn. Subdurals can present with failure to improve or fluctuating drowsiness. They either regress spontaneously or require surgical drainage but have a propensity to recur.

  ▸▸ ***Subdural haematoma pp 411-2***

Extradurals

Scan 'B' is a CT showing two very large haemorrhagic frontal extradurals with a third smaller localised extradural on the right. Extradurals usually present acutely, sometimes after a brief lucid interval where the patient awakens following loss of consciousness for anything from a few minutes to a few hours, then shows a rapidly deteriorating level of consciousness level often leading to death if untreated within a few hours.

NOTE
Haemorrhage into the extradural or subdural space acts as a space occupying lesion and contributes to raised intracranial pressure

3.1.4

- **Diffuse axonal injury**

The MRI scan shows extensive bilateral white matter damage to the frontal lobes which represents diffuse axonal injury (a.k.a. 'diffuse white matter damage'). This occurs in white matter tracts of the cerebral hemispheres, including the corpus callosum (leading to atrophy and diffuse ventricular enlargement), and the brainstem, particularly the cerebellar peduncles. Over the first 24-48 hours axons break up, forming 'retraction balls'.

Clinical findings will depend on the severity and extent of brain damage, and include:

- prolonged coma in the absence of a focal brain lesion
- severe cognitive impairment and personality change
- neurological signs, particularly from involvement of long tracts in the brain stem and cerebellar peduncles
- dysarthria
- possible quadriparesis and ataxia

⏩ ***pg 163, column 1***

3.1.5

- **Hydrocephalus**

The scan shows bilateral, lateral ventricular dilitation with periventricular oedema (slightly more pronounced in the left posterior horn), indicative of hydrocephalus.

The two processes that could lead to this presentation are:

- **Non-obstructive Hydrocephalus** ("ex-vacuo")
  - due to atrophy of surrounding white/grey matter
- **Obstructive hydrocephalus** ("normal pressure hydrocephalus")
  - due to blockage of free CSF circulation within the subarchnoid space, leading to raised intracranial pressure

It's likely that the clinical presentation and scan findings are due to obstructive (normal pressure) hydrocephalus. This leads to late deterioration in metal state months or years following a closed head injury, and is more likely to occur if there was substantial subarachnoid bleeding at the time of the injury.

Typical neuropsychiatric features include;

- deteriorating cognitive performance
- deteriorating personality change / behavioral problems
- increasing neurological problems in particular: gait disturbance and incontinence

Treatment

Ventriculo-peritoneal shunt may improve mental state and prevent further deterioration

⏩ ***pg 744***

NEUROPSYCHIATRIC SEQUELAE

The remaining sections in this module deal with the aetiological factors and clinical presentations of neuropsychiatric disorders in traumatic brain injury.The causes for the brain to be injured are varied (as section 3.1 highlighted) and the site damaged will govern much of the cognitive abnormalities observed. It is useful to consider the aetiological causes of psychiatric disorder under the categories of pre-traumatic (e.g. premorbid personality), peri-traumatic (e.g.degree and severity of brain damage) and post-traumatic (e.g. impact of injury to patient and others).

▸▸ ***Aetiology of psychiatric disability after head injury pp 172-82 and Categories of post-traumatic disorder pp 182-99***

You may wish to read more on these topics before moving on

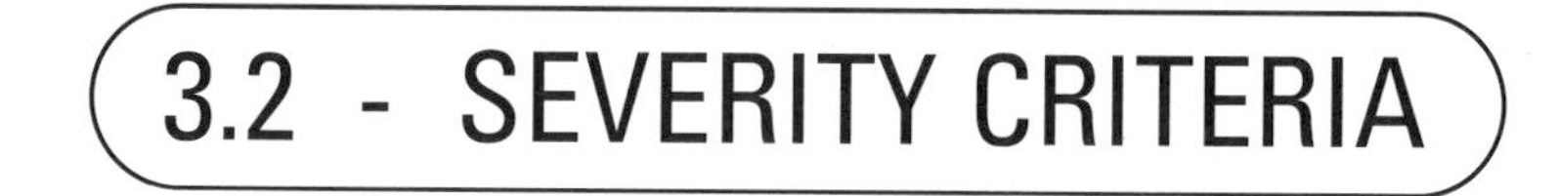

This section deals with the criteria of severity in head injury. Measuring severity has been found to be predictive of future cognitive disturbance.

▸▸ *Amnesic defects surrounding injury pp 169-71*
You may wish to read something on this topic before attempting the exercise

▶ PLAY THE VIDEO

Exercise 3.2

Excerpt 3.2 features Dr Fleminger interviewing an executive businessman in his 50's who sustained a head injury after falling 2m off a ladder. He's recorded in this excerpt talking about events that he can recall before and after the event. Keep in mind what the examiner is attempting to illustrate.

Watch the whole excerpt and then write answers to questions 3.2.1 - 3.2.2. Feedback is given over the page but try answering each question before looking

3.2.1
What severity criteria are elicited in this excerpt?
(which do you think is the best in terms of predicting the clinical outcome after head injury?)

3.2.2
What is this man's prognosis of returning to work as an executive?

3.2.1

There is no universally accepted classification of head injury severity. The excerpt highlighted two of the principle measures of severity, namely:

- **Duration of coma** (12 days)
- **Duration of post-traumatic amnesia - PTA** (4 weeks)

⏩ **Post-traumatic amnesia *pp 169-70***

Glasgow coma scale (GCS) is a third widely used grading system; it is usually measured on admission to casualty

⏩ ***p167***

- **Mild:** GCS 13-15;
  generally associated with a loss of consciousness
  <20min / PTA <24 hours
- **Moderate:** GCS 9-12;
  generally associated with a loss of consciousness
  <24 hours / PTA <1 week
- **Severe:** GCS 3-8;
  generally associated with a loss of consciousness
  >24 hours / PTA >1 week

Note in this man's case, the length of coma and duration of PTA may have been prolonged by sedation for ventilation. The excerpt also highlights a retrograde amnesia of 30-60 minutes

⏩ ***Retrograde amnesia pp 170-1 and Shrinkage of the RA pp 30 and 36***

3.2.2

Prognosis for work

Post Traumatic Amnesia (PTA) is the memory loss for events following the lesion and ends when there is a return of continuous registration of personal memory. Retrospective assessment is most accurate and it is regarded as the best predictor of cognitive dysfunction.

A PTA of 24 hours may be regarded as a watershed; below this full recovery can be expected, above this and some degree of cognitive impairment is expected. With a PTA of 4 weeks or more (as described in this man's history), a closed head injury is likely to be followed by invalidism extending over the greater part of a year (⏩ *p171 column 1*). The prognosis must be adjusted in relation to likely demands made upon the individual. The figures in table 7 (pg 171) are crude/overall estimates and do not take account of the complexity of the individual's pre-injury occupation/ vocation. People are less likely to be able to return to high level professional jobs. This might reflect damage to 'executive' systems resulting in impairments of self-monitoring, planning and organisational skills.

⏩ ***Cognitive impairment pp182-7 and Intellectual impairment pp 212-3 (treatment issues)***

You may wish to consolidate these points before moving onto the next section

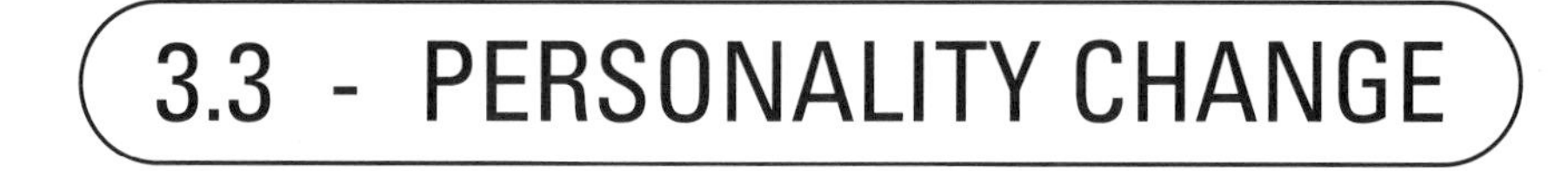

3.3 - PERSONALITY CHANGE

Head injury results in both physical and psychological trauma. The clinical picture is a reflection of the interplay between the brain injury (ie site affected, degree of damage etc) and the psychodynamic processes that follow. The consequences are often devastating and enduring. The behavioural and personality changes compromise some of the most difficult problems to re-dress, as the clinical picture is an admixture of accentuated previous traits and new behaviour never manifest before the insult.

Two exercises are given in this section that highlight these issues; the first based around a video excerpt and the second around a vignette and scan

▸▸ ***Change of personality pp 187-90***
This covers further details which you may wish to refer to during the next exercise

▶ PLAY THE VIDEO

Exercise 3.3

Excerpt 3.3 features Dr Fleminger interviewing a man who has suffered a very severe head injury. The patient was hit by a car while crossing the road. He was unconscious for about two days and the duration of post-traumatic amnesia was estimated as about two months. He is being interviewed about a year later having made an uneventful physical recovery from his injuries. The excerpt also features his daughter, seen separately, who gives an account of a dramatic change in his personality.

Watch the excerpt and then answer questions 3.3.1-3.3.3. Feedback is given over the page but try answering each question before looking

3.3.1
What key aetiological factors could have contributed to his presentation?

3.3.2
Do you think that the severity of his brain injury played a part?

3.3.3
What factors may have contributed to the increasing problems at home?

FEED BACK

3.3.1

Aetiological factors:

- **Brain damage to 'silent' regions of the brain**
  i.e. those not producing physical (neurological) deficits. These would contribute to the changes in his personsonality described by his daughter (i.e. disinhibition, motivational decline etc)
- **Pre-traumatic personality**
  This has a pathoplastic effect on the personality change observed following traumatic brain injury. His daughter describes accentuations in his previous traits.

  In general, anti-social personality traits pre-injury tend to be remarkably exacerbated by closed head injury. With open head injury, the personality change is much more dependent on localisation and is rarely seen if the injury doesn't involve the frontotemporal lobes.

  ▸▸ ***See pp 172-6***

3.3.2

Severity of brain injury:

- more severe injury is associated with personality change

3.3.3

Factors contributing to problems at home:

- **Patient factors**
  - **poor insight**
  - **nature of the personality change**

  Both issues will stretch the family's ability to cope

- **Secondary problems**
  - **financial difficulties from loss of income**
  - **family's response**

  This case highlights the morbid effects that brain injury has on relationships. As the family struggle to cope with the patient's unreasonableness, their stress increases and this will exacerbate his behavioral problems.

▸▸ ***Change of personality pp187-90***
re-read this if you need to before tackling the second part of this exercise

feedback

Exercise 3.3 (cont.) VIGNETTE

A 35 year old man presents with personality change and chaotic lifestyle 5 years after mild head injury when he was elbowed in the face and fell backwards and cracked his head on the floor. He had a convulsion on hitting the ground and was then unconscious for 5 minutes. He was in hospital for 5 days post injury and he was thought to have frontal lobes damage. You are informed that apart from being rather tired the only change noted in hospital was that he took part in some rather childish pranks; on one occasion he stripped naked on the ward. Also, he easily loses his temper, displays antisocial behaviour and appears unable to organise his life. Standard psychometry was normal (WAIS and WMS normal) but measures of executive function showed moderate to severe impairment. A CT brain scan was normal and his MRI is shown.

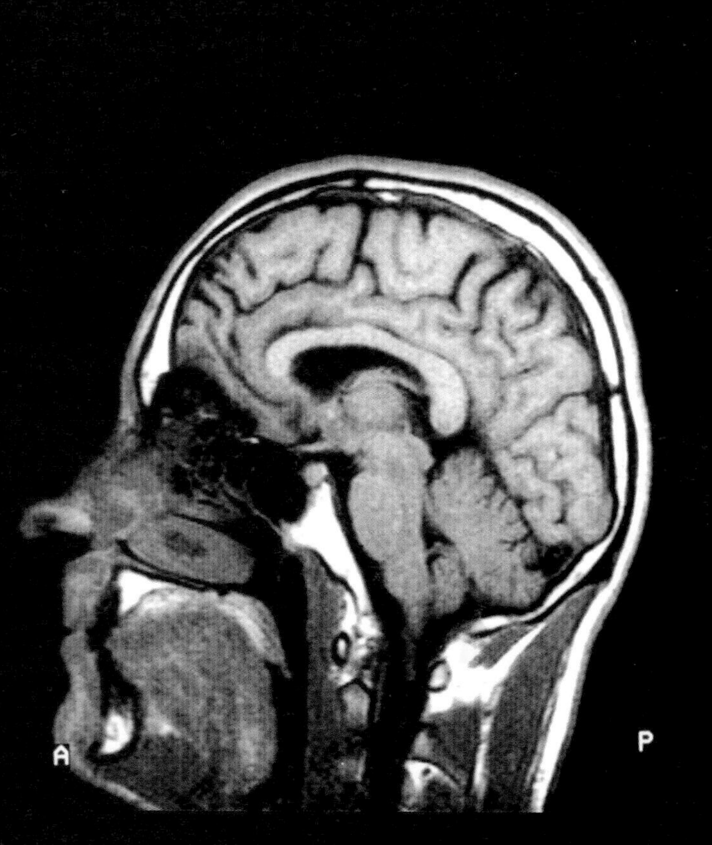

3.3.4
What frontal lobe injury is suggested by this man's presentation?

3.3.5
Are his symptoms typical of such an injury?

3.3.6
Are his immediate fits associated with a poor outcome?

3.4.7
What physical sign, associated with frontal lobe injury, might you be eager to enquire about?

3.3.4

- **Medial orbital injury of the frontal lobe**
  CT brain scans are much less sensitive than MRI. They are particularly poor at viewing the bone/brain interface where contusions are found - his MRI scan shows a contusion to the medial orbital area.

3.3.5

Symptoms:

- **Typical of frontal lobe syndrome - disinhibition, childish behaviour, lack of judgement etc.**
  Medial orbital frontal injury is particularly associated with antisocial personality change after traumatic brain injury and is a common site of traumatic injury.

3.3.6

Fits:

- **Immediate fits are not associated with a poor outcome**

3.3.7

Physical sign:

- **Anosmia** - serves as a risk factor for acquired antisocial personality disorder

▸▸ ***Personality change and behavioural disorder pp 213-4***
Further discussion on important treatment issues

feedback

3.4 - POST-CONCUSSIONAL SYNDROME

Also known as 'post-traumatic syndrome' this is an area of controversy, highlighting the interplay between organic and psychogenic factors in symptom formation. This section presents a brief clinical excerpt in which the patient describes some common symptoms.

▸▸ ***Neurotic disability and Post-traumatic syndrome pp 193-9***
You may wish to read further details before proceeding

▶ PLAY THE VIDEO

Exercise 3.4

Excerpt 3.4 features a woman who was hit on the right side of the head by a golf ball. She suffered brief loss of consciousness, not requiring admission to hospital. The interview takes place two years later.

Write down answers to the questions below, after you've viewed the excerpt. Feedback is given over the page but try answering each question before looking.

3.4.1
What symptoms of post-concussional syndrome does she describe?
(give at least three)

3.4.2
She has responded to cognitive behavioural therapy; what techniques may have been used?
(name three)

FEED BACK

3.4.1

Symptoms of post concussional syndrome:

Early:

- **Lethargy** (excessive tiredness)
- **Derealisation** ("in a dream")
- **Pain and headaches**
- **Diplopia**
- **Dizziness**

Late:

- **Mood swings**
- **Anxiety**
- **Memory and concentration difficulties**

3.4.2

Cognitive behavioural therapy techniques:

- **Anxiety management**
- **Graded return to activities**
- **Reattribution of symptoms**

▸▸ 196-9

If you need to, re-read the details on this condition before moving on

3.5 - PSYCHOSIS

Psychosis is both an early and late issue in the brain-injured patient. This section presents an brief interview to introduce an important phenomenon is this area.

Acute post-traumatic psychosis pp 168-9 and Psychosis pp190-2

You may wish to read up about the subject before tackling the exercise

PLAY THE VIDEO

Exercise 3.5

Excerpt 3.5 features an interview on the ward, between Dr Fleminger and a patient. The recording was made 2 months after a severe brain injury with bi-frontal contusions (not 16-18 weeks as the patient declares). The interview takes place at the Maudsley, London (UK)

Watch the video and answer question 3.5.1 before turning to the feedback

3.5.1

What would you call the phenomenon that he is describing?

FEEDBACK

3.5.1

- **Reduplicative paramnesia**
(also known as 'double orientation')

The patient acknowledges having had a head injury but maintains that this occurred in Italy, not the UK. He firmly believes that he remains in Italy and misidentifies cues around him, which serve to further support his delusion.

Delusions of misidentification may be observed early in the course of recovery and are often associated with more generalised disturbances of insight, judgement and disorientation.

▸▸ ***Reduplicative paramnesia pp 11-12***

Other psychotic phenomena are discussed in the references given at the start of the section. Re-read these if necessary.

3.6 - PSYCHOLOGICAL COMPLICATIONS

Sometimes the condition that your patient presents with is extremely puzzling. Differentiating the contributions of physical and psychological factors on the clinical picture may be hard, as this next exercise demonstrates.

PLAY THE VIDEO

Exercise 3.6

Excerpt 3.6 features a man in his 30's presenting with progressive deterioration in level of independence and cognition 3 years following head injury. He is now said to be entirely dependent on his wife, does very little and talks in a childlike manner. His Glasgow coma scale score on admission was 12 and it is likely that he lost consciousness for no more than a few minutes. His PTA was never assessed and it is not possible to assess it now. He never had a brain scan at the time of the injury and his present MRI brain scan shows no abnormality. He has very poor performance on formal neuropsychological testing. All other investigations are normal, except for observations on the ward which indicates that his performance deteriorates after weekend leave. Staff note that his wife is reluctance to have him stay in hospital for very long. Despite performing very badly on neuropsychological testing, he is able at times to play complex board games (e.g.scrabble) with other patients, and win. The patient is pursuing compensation for his injury.

Write down answers to questions 3.6.1-3.6.2 after watching the excerpt. Feedback is given over the page but try answering each question before looking

3.6.1
Do these findings rule out a significant brain injury in this man?

3.6.2
What do you think is the likely explanation for the majority of his disability and how might you manage his case?

3.6.1

- **Severe head injury is NOT ruled out**
  Some investigators suggest that diffuse axonal injury (DAI) may not be detectable in certain cases even with MRI. Also, an independent presenile dementing process should be excluded

3.6.2

Likely explanation for the majority of his disability:

- **Psychogenic reaction/ hysterical dissociative state**
  The excerpt shows how the patient can clearly comprehend what is being asked but responds in bizarre ways, with an exaggerated desire to please. His cognitive errors are variable. But note, he shows perseveration when he writes down numbers (1 to 10) when asked to write his address; this may indicate organic pathology.

Other factors contributing to his presentation include:

- **Compensation claim**
- **Other secondary gain** (as yet unknown)
- **Wife's maladaptive response**
- **Anxiety response to mild cognitive impairment**

A way of managing this kind of presentaion would be:

- **Therapeutic optimism**
- **Engage in rehabilitation programme** (excuse to get better)
- **Consider limiting contact with wife**
- **Marital therapy**
- **Speedy resolution of any compensation claim**

see also:

- ***Case vignette pg 193***
  highlights similar themes
- ***Rehabilitation units pp 215-6***
- ***Medicolegal considerations pp 207-11***

M3 SUMMARY

We've got to the end of module three.

The key learning points have been the need to consider the following; the individual (their traits and dispositions), the nature and circumstance of the injury and the physical and psychological sequelae.

Michelle V Lambert

MODULE 4

Epilepsy

CONTENTS

aims

This module aims to:

- give a brief overview of the subject, focusing on aspects of epilepsy that are of particular relevance to psychiatrists
- stress that distinguishing 'true' seizures from 'pseudo' seizures is extremely difficult, and that the two may co-exist
- highlight the factors contributing to psychiatric co-morbidity in people with epilepsy

objectives

At the end of the module you should be able to:

- understand that there are different seizure types and epilepsy syndromes, which have important implications for management
- be aware of the phenomena encountered in complex partial seizures
- give examples of conditions that give rise to epilepsy and the differential diagnosis of attacks

PLAY THE VIDEO

Introduction 4.0

Excerpt 4.0 features Dr Lambert and Professor Goldberg discussing three areas of the subject; the value in distinguishing syndrome and seizure types, key features in the history that help diagnostic assessment and psychiatric co-morbidity

Play the video and stop when prompted

Varieties of epilepsy pp 237-42

Epilepsy is a complex disorder, difficult for both patients and doctors to understand. It is a condition in which seizures occur, usually spontaneously. Seizures are stereotyped, intermittent disturbances of brain function and are caused by a number of factors. You may wish to read the introductory paragraphs to chapter 7 and the varieties of epilepsy before tackling section 4.1 which looks at different clinical presentations

4.1 - SEIZURES & SYNDROMES

We start with a look at the importance of differentiating seizure and syndrome types. The exercise in this section presents a number of excerpts of patients having epileptic seizures. Before tackling the exercise, famalarise yourself with the classifications below.

EPILEPTIC SEIZURES

- classified by onset (using clinical and EEG information)

- **Generalised epilepsy;**
  Absence ('petit mal'), Primary generalised ('tonic-clonic'), Myoclonic, Tonic, Clonic, Atonic and Atypical
- **Partial epilepsy** (± secondary generalisation)
  Simple partial seizures - 'auras'
  Sensory, motor, psychic or autonomic ▸▸ ***pp 249-52***
  - consciousness is retained

  Complex partial seizures - 'psychomotor seizures'
  Fugues, automatisms and twilight state ▸▸ ***pp 252-9 & 296-8***
  - consciousness is disturbed at onset

EPILEPTIC SYNDROMES

- classified by aetiology and characteristics of the disorder

- **Idiopathic (primary)**
- **Symptomatic (secondary)**
- **Cryptogenic**
- **Special syndromes**

▶ P L A Y T H E V I D E O

Exercise 4.1

The excerpts 4.1.1 - 4.1.4 show patients having seizures. *Pause between each excerpt to write a response to the question below. Feedback is given over the page but try giving an answer for each excerpt before looking*

What type of epilepsy is being shown in each excerpt?
(give reasons for your answers)

4.1.1 Man in kitchen, making a cup of tea
4.1.2 Boy playing with toys
(same seizure with and without telemetry)
4.1.3 Two patients showing the same seizure
(with telemetry)
4.1.4 Man reading, followed by a boy taking a hot bath
(both highlight a rare syndrome)

FEED BACK

4.1.1

- **Complex partial seizure of supplementary motor area origin with automatism.**
  - disturbance of consciousness & automatic fumbling without awareness
  - 'fencing' posture at the onset is typical of seizures arising in the supplementary motor area

    ⏩ ***Focal epilepsy pp 239-41 & Frontal seizures pp 249-50***

4.1.2

- **Absence** ('petit mal') **seizure**
  - abrupt onset/offset - looks blank, blinks and then resumes normal activities
  - EEG characteristic

    ⏩ ***Generalised epilepsy pp 238-9***

4.1.3

- **Myoclonic jerks**

    ⏩ ***pp 238-9***

4.1.4

- **Reflex epilepsy**
  - the first case shows a man having a generalised seizure precipitated by reading.
  - the second case shows a boy having a partial seizure precipitated by hot water.

    ⏩ ***Other forms of epilepsy pp 241-2***

NOTE

- *Your patient may suffer from more than one seizure type*
- *Certain anti-epileptic drugs are only licensed for particular seizure types*
- *A syndrome does not necessarily have a common aetiology and prognosis, as highlighted below:*

  Idiopathic (primary)
  - genetic cause with less neurological dysfunction
  - usually normal background inter-ictal activity
  - seizures relatively self-limited and responsive to medication

  Symptomatic (secondary)
  - associated with abnormal neurological development or cerebral disease,
  - inter-ictal EEGs shows slow background activity.
  - seizures less likely to remit spontaneously
  - variable response to medication.

  Cryptogenic
  - aetiology is as yet unknown
  - no well-defined electroclinical features are found

  Special syndromes
  - e.g. reflex epilepsy and febrile convulsion

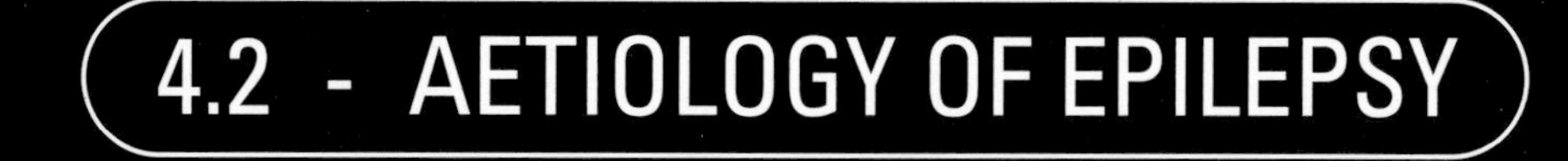

4.2 - AETIOLOGY OF EPILEPSY

Epilepsy is a symptom; the aetiological causes are multiple. The aim here is to consider those causes.

▸▸ ***Prevalence and aetiology pp 242-8***
The topic is covered in detail on thes pages, but try the exercise first before consulting the text

---

Exercise 4.2

Questions 4.2.1 and 4.2.2 relate to the two scans of conditions that give rise to seizures.
Write an answer to the questions for each and then in question 4.2.3, see how many other conditions you can think of that may lead to seizure activity.

4.2.1 (Scan A)
What important brain malformation do you think gave rise to this individual's epilepsy?

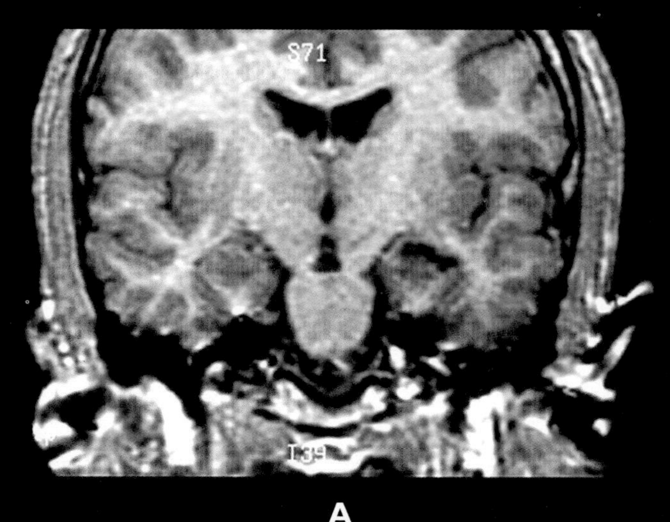

A

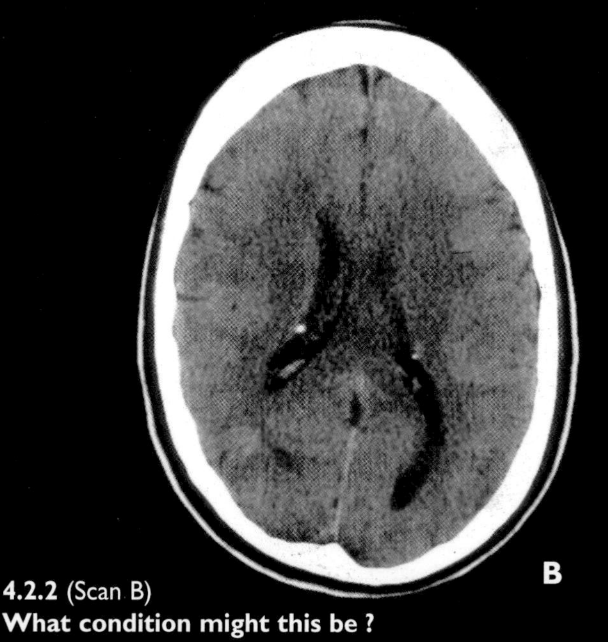

B

4.2.2 (Scan B)
What condition might this be ?

4.2.3
List other causes of epilepsy, stating their likely ages of onset.
(Try to give at least eight)

4.2.1

- **Mesial temporal sclerosis**
  Scan 'A' is an MRI T1 weighted coronal slice showing a change in tissue within the anterior hippocampus, far worse on the left than the right. This is the commonest brain malformation causing epilepsy
  Onset: usually early (infancy/early childhood), but may develop in adulthood

4.2.2

- **Tuberous Sclerosis**
  Scan 'B' is a CT scan showing a high-density lesion (pearly white nodules - probably calcified) on appendymal surface of lateral vetricle with slight atrophy, which is a characteristic finding in this condition. It is a foetal developmental abnormality with a triad of mental subnormality, epilepsy and adenoma
  Onset: early (infancy/early childhood)
  ▸▸ *pp 701-3*

4.2.3
Other causes:

- **Congenital brain malformations**
  Examples include porencephaly; arteriovenous malformations (e.g. Sturge-Weber); cortical dysgenesis; dysembryoplastic neuroepithelial tumour (DNET)
  Onset: early (infancy/early childhood)
- **Genetic**
  Autosomal dominant or chromosomal
  Onset: usually early childhood
- **Birth injury**
  Onset: usually early
- **Head Injury - post traumatic**
  Onset: Usually adulthood, seizures usually begin within 3 years of injury, but 1/5 have onset >4 years post head injury
- **Post-infective**
  Examples include cerebral infections (i.e. encephalitis, meningitis, cerebral abscess, tuberculoma, neurosyphilis and paracystic cysts) or secondary to systemic infections resulting in pyrexia and febrile convulsions
  Onset; any age (except febrile convulsions which occur in infancy)
- **Cerebrovascular disease**
  Secondary to cerebral arteriosclerosis, hypertensive encephalopathy, cerebral embolus, thrombosis or haemorrhage
  Onset: usually late adult years
- **Cerebral tumours**
  Following primary and secondary neoplasia
  Onset: any age
- **Degenerative disorders**
  Examples include Alzheimer's disease and Lipoidoses
  Onset: childhood and later life
- **Drugs, toxins and metabolic disorders**
  Examples include uraemia, hypocalcaemia and overdose
  Onset: any age

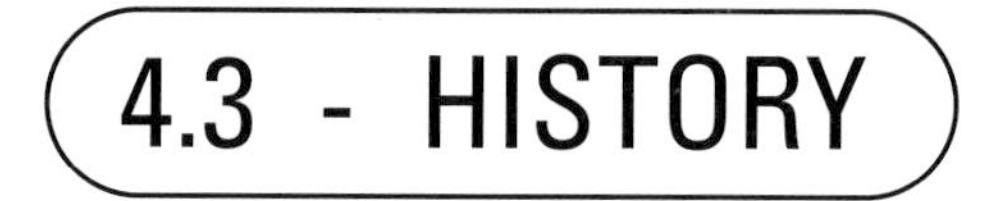

4.3 - HISTORY

In order to make a diagnosis of epilepsy it is essential to take a clear, detailed history from the patient and ideally an informant who has witnessed the attack. Clinically it helps to distinguish seizure related manifestations (prodromal, peri-ictal, and post-ictal periods) from interictal phenomena. The prodrome tends to be a non-specific 'warning' (apprehension/ dullness) varying from hours to days.

The exercise here aims to highlight an interviewing technique that covers these manifestations and phenomena. Given that the patient is being interviewed alone, an enquiry is made into what he knows about his seizures from what he is told happens during an attack.

PLAY THE VIDEO

Exercise 4.3

Excerpt 4.3 features Dr Toone taking a history from a man who has epilepsy.

When you've seen the excerpt, attempt the following questions. Feedback is given overleaf but write something down in you answer book before looking.

4.3.1
What type of epilepsy do you think the patient describes?
(give reasons for your answer)

4.3.2
What additional information (if any) would support your diagnosis?
(give at least six)

4.3.1

- **Partial epilepsy with secondary generalisation**
  - simple partial seizure (aura) with feeling of panic
    (note: the patient is incorrectly using the term 'petit mal')
  - prodrome lasting several days during which he experiences a feeling of unreality (depersonalisation - "a trance-like state")
  - progression into a secondarily generalised seizure
    This is not described but he does give a good history of the witness report. His right arm and leg go into extension/abduction, followed by jerking of all limbs, loss of consciousness, tongue biting, urinary incontintence and self-injury. Sometimes there is no progression of the seizure.

Focus: dominant temporal lobe

An onset with right arm and leg jerking, aphasia and post-ictal dysphasia would be compatable with a focus in the dominant left hemisphere (note that the patient is right handed). The most likely focus is in the temporal lobe given that he experiences an aura, motionless stare (motor arrest), aphasia at onset, autonomic changes (pallor) and post ictal confusion (with a 10-15 minute delay in fully regaining consciousness), and post-ictal dysphasia ("talking garbage") His slow recovery, lack of nocturnal attacks and lack of seizure clustering would go against a diagnosis of frontal seizures although the motor onset - right arm and leg (dystonic posturing) - would support consideration for such attacks.

4.3.2

Additional information

- **Physical examination**; interictal examination is usually normal but the post-ictal examination may reveal localising signs such as Todd's paresis ▸▸ *pg 240*
- **History from informant**
- **Family history of epilepsy**
- **Early personal/developmental history**; including perinatal injuries/complications, early developmental milestones; febrile convulsions (number/duration and focal features); head injury or infection.
- **Drug/alcohol misuse/dependence/withdrawal**
- **Other medical illnesses/medication**
- **EEG**: routine +/- sleep activation
- **Neuroimaging**; indicated if there are:
  - localising signs
  - seizures arising in the neonatal period or after the age of 20
  - secondary symptoms - e.g. Todd's paralysis/dysphasias
  - focal seizures, with or without focal CNS signs
  - treatment resistance
  - relapse of previously well-controlled seizures

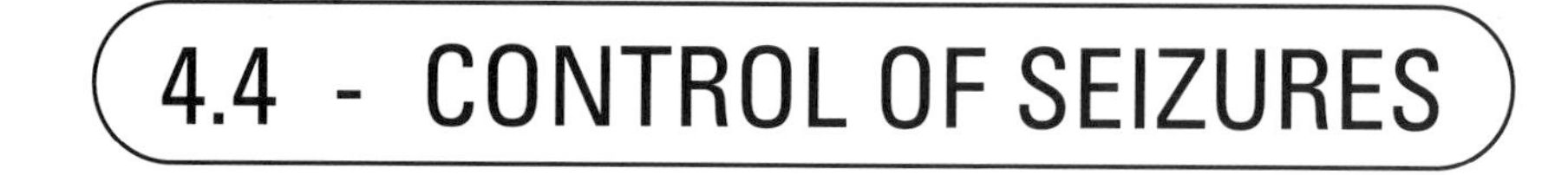

4.4 - CONTROL OF SEIZURES

In addition to pharmacological seizure control it is important to enquire about whether your patient can exert any voluntary control over their seizures. The exercise in this section starts with an introduction to the topic and then shows an interview with two young women who describe strategies they employ to attempt to control their attacks. The capacity to control seizures in no way means that the patient doesn't suffer from them.

▸▸ *Treatment pp 298-314*

The section on psychological and social aspects of management is particularly relevant to the following exercise. You may wish to also read up about anticonvulsant medication and surgical treatments, which will not be further discussed in this module.

▶ PLAY THE VIDEO

Exercise 4.4

Excerpt 4.4 features Dr Fenwick and Professor Goldberg, discussing strategies for controlling certain types of seizures. Their discussion is followed by two women describing their experiences of adopting these straegies.

Write down an answer to question 4.4.1 when you have seen the whole excerpt. Feedback is given over the page but try answering each question before looking

4.4.1

What strategies, discussed in the excerpts, may be used to control seizures?

4.4.1
Cognitive - behavioural techniques discussed:
(These are especially useful with partial seizures which have a prodromal warning)

- **Define the aura**
  Encourage your patient to reach a more detailed understanding and recognition of their simple partial seizures (auras). These herald the seizure onset where consciousness is retained. If a patient can learn to recognise the signs, then they may have a chance to counter a full-blown convulsion

- **Opposing movements**
  Used if the seizure is motor
  (e.g. pressing the hand back as it goes into flexion)

- **Distraction**
  Used if the seizure is sensory
  (e.g. counting backwards or visualisation of a plesant scene)

- **Symptom diary**
  Identify stresses and precipitants to the seizures

▸▸ ***Behavioural treatments pp 308-9***

4.5 - DIFFERENTIAL DIAGNOSIS

Cerebral function can be intermittently disturbed by a number of conditions that can mimic epilepsy. Here, we look at some examples.

▸▸ ***Investigations and differential diagnosis pp 286-98***
These pages cover the topic in detail, but try the exercise first

Exercise 4.5

4.5.1

A 52 year old businessman develops episodes of loss of consciousness without warning. He was previously well except for a history of hypertension and occasional palpitations and shortness of breath when exercising. Witnesses described that he suddenly falls to the ground, looking pale, is unconsciousness for several minutes, then regains consciousness. At times there have been reports suggestive of convulsions during these episodes.

What is your diagnosis ?

(Give your reasons. Don't turn over for the answer until you've tried the next example)

4.5.2

A 43 year old woman presents with a history of having one episode of loss of consciousness during the night, 5 weeks ago. She woke at 3am, feeling unwell, with stomach pain and nausea. She then went into the bathroom and after a few minutes, her husband went after her to check whether she needed help. She remembered feeling ill and very tired and the surroundings appeared distorted. She felt light headed, dizzy and very hot. She experienced a ringing in her ears and "everything went black". As her husband walked into the bathroom, he discovered that she appeared very pale and was collapsing to the ground. He immediately grabbed her and held her upright. However, she then lost consciousness. Her husband then noticed twitching of all limbs and she was incontinent of urine. He placed her on the bathroom floor and phoned for an ambulance. A few minutes later she regained consciousness, but felt unwell complaining of having a headache, feeling hot, perspiring and experiencing nausea.

What is your diagnosis ?

(give your reasons)

4.5.3

What other conditions would you consider in your differential for epilepsy?

4.5.1

- **Cardiac arrhythmia (Stoke Adams attacks)**
  - sudden onset
  - history of hypertension, palpitations and shortness of breath
  - stress

Epilepsy should be a differential diagnosis as these attacks may be secondary anoxic seizures. If the episode of loss of consciousness is less than 1 minute, an arrhythmia is more likely. EEG telemetry with an ECG lead would help you distinguish.

4.5.2

- **Vaso-vagal attack (faint)**
  - patient felt unwell before the attack
  - gradual onset of episode with autonomic changes (e.g. nausea, dizziness and pallor), ringing in ears and visual disturbance.
  - gradual collapse and rapid recovery when supine, followed by feeling hot and perspiring

Twitching occurred, which may be irregular myoclonic jerking, which occurs during syncope especially when not supine. Incontinence is rare but may happen especially if the bladder is full, such as during the night

4.5.3

Other differentials

Cardiac

- Micturition syncope
- Postural hypotension

Metabolic

- Hypoglycaemia
- Hypocalcaemia
- Hyperventilation
- Drug overdose

Neurological

- Transient Ischaemic Attacks
- Vertebrobasilar ischaemia
- Migraine
- Transient Global Amnesia
- Narcolepsy/cataplexy
- Paroxysmal choreoathetosis and hyperekplexia ('startle disease')

Psychiatric

- Dissociative disorders e.g. 'Pseudoseizures'
- Panic attacks
- Night terrors
- Somnambulism
- Breath holding attacks
- Transient acute organic reactions due to other causes
- Aggressive outbursts ('episodic dyscontrol')

▸▸ ***Investigations and differential diagnosis pp 286-98***

PSYCHIATRIC CO-MORBIDITY

The rest of this module will now look at the psychiatric co-morbidity of epilepsy.

Aetiology of psychiatric disorder in people with epilepsy

■ **Epilepsy factors**

- aetiology of epilepsy e.g. genetic, head injury etc
- age of onset and duration of epilepsy
- seizure or syndrome type e.g. localisation of focus
- increase (clustering) of seizures and change in severity
- cessation of seizures (i.e.'forced normalisation')

■ **Iatrogenic factors**

- type of antiepileptic drugs
- number of antiepileptic drugs
- serum level of antiepileptic drugs
- secondary effects of antiepileptic drug e.g. hormonal, serum folate deficiency
- effects of surgery

■ **Psychosocial factors**

- fear of seizures - unpredictability and lack of control
- stigma, discrimination and rejection
- adjustment to epilepsy - grief reaction
- overprotection e.g. from family and friends
- social support/isolation/occupational issues/driving status

Disorders commonly associated with epilepsy

All psychiatric disorders are encountered in people with epilepsy but the following list highlights some of the salient examples related to epilepsy:

- **Somatoform disorder**
  - Dissociative disorder - Pseudoseizure

- **Anxiety disorder**
  - Panic disorder
  - Obsessional Compulsive Disorder

- **Affective disorder**
  - Depressive reaction/feelings
  - Depressive Illness
  - Inter-ictal Dysphoric Disorder (IDD)

- **Psychosis**
  - Brief Interictal Psychosis
  - Chronic Interictal Psychosis (Schizophrenia-like psychosis of epilepsy, SLPE)
  - Post-ictal psychosis (PIP)

- **Personality disorder**
  - Religiosity/ Hypergraphia/ Viscosity
  - Sexual Dysfunction

- **Disorders of impulse control**
  - Anger/irritability
  - Drug/alcohol abuse

▸▸ ***Pschiatric disability among persons with epilepsy pp 259-86***

You may wish to refer to this reading during the next sections

4.6 - PSEUDOSEIZURES

There are many pseudonyms for pseudoseizures; psychogenic seizures, non epileptic attack disorder, non epilepic seizures and nonepileptic seizure like events. In psychogenic pseudoseizures, there is a change of consciousness or behaviour that is not due to a physiological cause or ictal/postictal events. There are important medical and psychosocial reasons for identifying patients with pseudoseizures, including avoiding the use of unnecessary and toxic anti-epileptic medication (especially in women of childbearing age) and avoiding the stigma and medicolegal implications of a diagnosis of epilepsy. Types of 'attacks' have been described including; 'swooning' (apparently unconscious with no convulsion), 'tantrums' (dramatic thrashing) and 'abreaction' (initial overbreathing then convulsions with arching and pelvic thrusting). Always obtain a collateral history from an informant, focusing on a clear description of the attacks along with an evaluation of current stresses and premorbid level of functioning. Pseudoseizures usually serve a function - they may be an expression of emotional needs or help the patient cope with/ escape from emotional difficulties. A clear, detailed account of the first episode may give clues as to its aetiology.

▸▸ ***Epilepsy versus pseudoseizures pp 292-4***
This gives further details on the topic

▶ PLAY THE VIDEO

Exercise 4.6

Excerpt 4.6 features Dr Toone and Professor Goldberg discussing the difficulties in making a distinction between pseudoseizures and true seizures. Strategies used in helping those presenting with pseudoseizures are also discussed. Excerpts 4.6.1 - 4.6.3 then show you three different patients having attacks.

After the introduction, play each excerpt, writing down an answer to the following question. Feedback is given over the page but try answering each question before looking

Do you think the condition shown is an epileptic seizure or a pseudoseizure?
(give reasons for your answers)

4.6.1 Woman on floor
(this attack has lasted over 15 minutes)

4.6.2 Man in bed
(ignore the television commentary)

4.6.3 Woman spinning
(two presentations of the same attack are shown)

4.6.1

- **Pseudoseizure**
  - dramatic thrashing with writhing and flailing movements
  - long duration with no cyanosis

4.6.1

- **Frontal lobe (complex partial) seizure, of supplementary motor area origin**
  - abrupt onset, brief duration (normally <30sec)
  - disturbance of consciousness and speech (vocalising)
  - complex, bizarre behaviour with bilateral clapping and bed slapping
  - post-ictal confusion and automatism (fumbling with leads)

» pp 249-50

4.6.1

- **Pseudoseizure**
  - very bizzare, stereotyped movement (praying)
  - tonic extension of limbs, followed by getting up and spinning

NOTE

A complex partial siezure of frontal lobe origin is a differential in both the examples of pseudoseizure shown here. You would need to do prolactin levels (baseline and within 20 mins of attack » p290) and EEG telemetry to confidently differentiate their presentations

Pointers suggesting a pseudoseizure was more likely include:

- **Demographics and background**
  - more common after the age of ten, women more than men
  - history of abuse (e.g. sexual)
  - failed response to antiepileptic medication or sudden loss of seizure control in patient previously well-maintained on medication
  - co-existing psychiatric disorders
- **Precipitant**
  - strong emotion or environmental stress (also capable of inducing real seizures)
  - onset and context
  - evolve gradually, usually in the presence of an audience
- **Duration, symptomatology and observed behaviour**
  - prolonged, without cyanosis, usually running a variable course
  - based on a model of epilepsy, but doesn't conform to any recognised type showing atypical sequencing (e.g. intermittent, arrhythmic, out-of-phase jerking) and variability between episodes
  - struggling with staff, resisting eye-opening and avoidance reaction shown to noxious stimuli
  - sudden offset with rapid return to alert, responsive state, often accompanyied by crying
  - urinary incontinence, tongue biting and self-injury do occur

Management:

- operant conditioning- attempt not to 'reward' seizure
- slowly withdraw anticonvulsant medication
- treat co-morbid conditions

4.7 - ANXIETY DISORDERS

The condition of ictal anxiety and panic attacks are often difficult to differentiate clinically.

▸▸ ***Neurosis pp 275-7***
You may wish to familiarise yourself with the detail of this topic before tackling this exercise

PLAY THE VIDEO

Exercise 4.7

Excerpt 4.7 features Dr Lambert interviewing a young woman who describes her experiences of ictal anxiety and panic attacks. The woman is 22 years old and is right handed. She developed episodes of loss of consciousness 5 years ago, diagnosed as partial epilepsy with secondary generalisation. Her birth and development were normal with no history of febrile convulsions. There was no significant past psychiatric history and the family history was negative for epilepsy but positive for depression. A year after her initial diagnosis, she underwent a 7cm left temporal lobectomy for suspected Rasmussen's encephalitis (progressive neurological dysfunction and aphasia), after MRI studies showed a progressive left hemisphere lesion. For 18 months she remained seizure free but clusters of generalised tonic-clonic seizures resumed, which are now starting to be controlled. During the post-operative period she also developed symptoms of panic.

Watch the excerpt and then write down an answer to question 4.7.1. Feedback is given over the page but try answering the question before looking at the answer

4.7.1
How can you distinguish between her panic attacks and her seizures ?
(mention at least 4 points of difference; state how each might help you)

FEEDBACK

4.7.1

This example illustrates the difficulty in distinguishing between panic attacks and epilepsy, both for the clinicain and patient. Often the two co-exist. A self re-inforcing situation may occur where the panic induced hyperventilation may precipitate a seizure and fear of having a seizure may result in the development of an anxiety disorder. The patient in this excerpt can identify that the panic attacks lack the ictal sensation of "somebody coming up behind" and she retains consciousness. Other than this, to her, the two are subjectively indistinguishable. The 'post-ictal' features of drowsiness and dysphasia help to make a diagnosis of ictal panic. An increase in her anticonvulsant medication reduced the number of episodes suggesting that they were epileptic in origin, but there are many factors contributing to her anxiety disorder that would still need to be addressed.

The following features help you differentiate between panic attacks and epilepsy:

- **Onset**
  - anxiety: sudden onset (may be unexpected)
  - seizure: may also start rapidly, but often following a warning
- **Symptoms**
  - if a patient experiences psychic simple partial seizures they may get feelings of fear and dissociation (derealisation/depersonalisation) very similar to a panic attack. Similarly, an autonomic simple partial seizure would mimic the autonomic arousal of a panic attack.
  - alteration in consciousness and localising post-ictal signs (e.g. aphasia) would distinguish
- **Duration**
  - panic attacks tend to last longer
- **Termination**
  - fatigue and confusion with epilepsy, whereas a full, rapid recovery (often with crying) with panic attacks
- **Investigations**
  - EEG may show epileptiform activity in the temporal lobe
  - MRI may show temporal lobe pathology in patients with epilepsy
- **Treatment**
  - seizures tend to respond to anticonvulsants
  - antidepressants may help panic attacks but exacerbate epilepsy

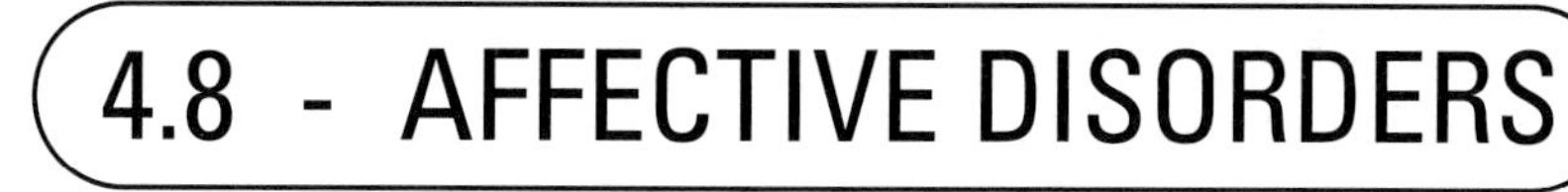

4.8 - AFFECTIVE DISORDERS

Distinguishing depressive reactions, periodic dysphoria and affective disorders is complex in people with epilepsy. The exercise here presents a case vignette to highlight some of these themes.

▸▸ ***Affective disturbance pp285-6***

You may wish to read further details on this topic before tackling the exercise

Exercise 4.8 VIGNETTE

A 30 year old man had a normal birth and development. He was average at school. There was no history of febrile convulsions, head injuries or cerebral infections. There was no family history of epilepsy, and the only psychiatric history was that his maternal grandmother committed suicide. He was first diagnosed as having epilepsy at the age of 5, when he had nocturnal tonic-clonic seizures. His daytime attacks begin with a warning consisting of a whistling/humming sensation in his head. Then his lips go white, he stares and fiddles with things using both hands and wanders about. He has no recollection of the attacks, only being aware that they have occurred when he finds himself in an unexpected place. He was treated with phenytoin throughout his childhood and early adult life and on this medication, he only experienced seizures 3-4 times a year. However, he developed gum hypertrophy and was switched on to carbamazepine. His seizure frequency increased to attacks every 1-2 weeks and Lamotrigine was added; this combination helped reduce the frequency of seizures.

At the age of 29, he was working as a clerk and was under pressure from his manager, who was critical of him. He suddenly began to feel depressed, irritable, nervous, tense and anxious. He developed derealisation with things around him appearing "different", and he did not recognise members of his household. He found it difficult to concentrate on watching television and at times thought that the programmes may have been referring to him. He began misinterpreting what people said to him. "Violent thoughts" started going through his head and he became preoccupied with knives, and the words "kill, stab" kept going through his mind although he tried to stop himself from thinking them. He started doing things in a repetitive way, despite realising that it was "silly". He was referred to a neuropsychiatrist. When seen, he brought four A4 pages of information with him, typed with small print explaining in intricate detail the recent events, including verbatim accounts of his conversations with his neurologist. He complained of being tearful, having initial insomnia, early morning wakening, reduced appetite and having a loss of enjoyment in things.

4.8.1
What kind of epilepsy do you think he has, and why?
4.8.2
What medication might be suitable for this kind of seizure?
4.8.3
What is your psychiatric diagnosis?
4.8.4
How would you treat him?
4.8.5
How far is the risk of suicide increased in this patient?

4.8.1

- **Partial seizures with secondary generalisations**
  - warning (simple partial seizures)
  - progression to a complex partial seizure with automatisms (fiddling with his hands and wandering)
  - Initial seizure would be compatible with a secondary generalised seizure
  - onset of staring suggests a temporal lobe focus, as does the history of automatisms.

4.8.2

Medications for partial seizures include:

- **Carbamazepine, Phenytoin, Valproate, Lamotrigine**

4.8.3

- **Moderate depressive disorder**

He describes several features; derealisation, obsessional ruminations of the phrase - "kill, stab" - and compulsions to perform rituals repetitively, ideas of reference with retained insight. The detailed A4 manuscript would be compatible with the behaviour of someone with an obsessional personality (often reported in patients with temporal lobe epilepsy). The onset appeared to be quite sudden, but this has been reported as typical of depression occurring in people with epilepsy. Depression appears to occur more commonly in patients with complex partial seizures, especially of left temporal lobe origin, and the severity of depression relates to the duration of epilepsy. Note, also, that depression is more common with phenobarbitone, phenytoin and vigabatrin.

4.8.4

Treatment options:

- **Improve seizure control and rationalise anticonvulsants** (monotherapy when possible)
- **Supportive psychotherapy for depressive reactions**
- **Antidepressants**
  - all antidepressants may lower the seizure threshold to some degree
  - there is little evidence that the newer drugs are strongly proconvulsant
  - start at a low dose and gradually increase to therapeutic levels
  - consider a serotonin reuptake inhibitor (SSRI) to treat the obsessional ruminations in addition to the depression.
- **ECT**
  - not contraindicated in epilepsy

4.8.5

- **Suicide**

There is a considerable risk of suicide in people with epilepsy, especially when the focus is in the temporal lobe; the rate has been reported to be increased by a factor of 25 (» *pg 286*). This patient has a family history of suicide, a stressful job and is currently depressed, therefore should be regarded as a high risk. Consideration should be given to dispensing his medication to a family member who could monitor the number of tablets he takes.

4.9 - PSYCHOSIS

This section deals with the confusing territory of epileptic psychosis. Again, a case vignette has been chosen to highlight the salient themes.

▸▸ ***Psychosis pp 277-84***
You may wish to familarise yourself with the topic before tackling this exercise

---

Exercise 4.9 VIGNETTE

A 29 year old ambidextrous man developed epilepsy at the age of 17. His only family history of epilepsy is of one paternal cousin, although no details are known. There is no family psychiatric history. His birth and early development were normal, in particular he did not experience any febrile convulsions and achieved average results in his school exams. He worked as a clerical officer and denies abuse of alcohol or other psychoactive substances.

His epilepsy initially started nocturnally, with generalised tonic clonic seizures. Since then, he has developed different kinds of seizures, occurring during the daytime. He experiences a warning of déjà vu or a "feeling of warmth" rising in his epigastrium accompanied by facial flushing. During other episodes he may talk "rubbish" but tends to repeat the phrase "I can see you, but you can't see me". These episodes only last seconds but occurred over 10 times a month. He also experiences generalised tonic-clonic seizures without warnings, approximately 3-4 times a month. His MRI scan was normal, but a PET scan showed 16% reduction in FDG uptake in the right temporal lobe. His psychometric testing (Weschler Adult Intelligence Score, WAIS) showed a full scale IQ of 85, verbal IQ of 94 and a performance IQ of 78

Feedback is given over the page but try answering each question first

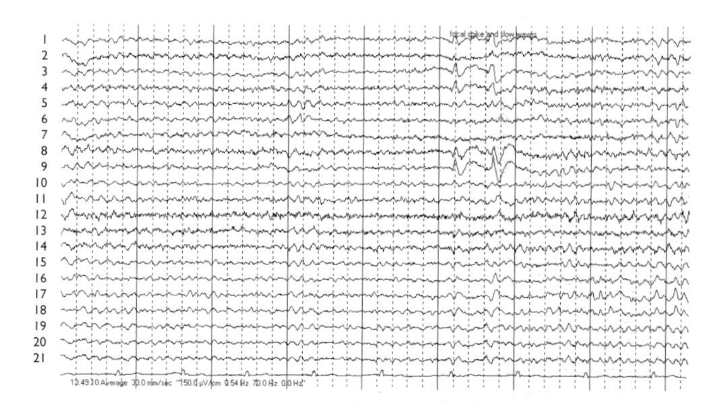

This was his EEG, montage Common Average Reference (see module 2, pg 32)

4.9.1
What kind of seizures do you think he experiences?

4.9.2
Comment on his EEG

4.9.3
Is his verbal-performance discrepancy significant & what does it suggest?

4.9.1
Seizure types:

- **Simple partial seizures (SPS): rising epigastric feeling, déjà vu**
- **Complex partial seizures: talking "rubbish"**
- **Secondary generalised seizures**

The most likely focus would be the temporal or frontal lobe. The SPS of déjà vu and a rising epigastric sensation accompanied by the autonomic symptom of facial flushing, would be compatible with the temporal lobe. The stereotyped speech automatisms suggest involvement of the right temporal lobe (contrasting with the post-ictal dysphasia which implicates the left temporal lobe). However, generalised seizures originating in the frontal lobe often occur nocturnally, and the history of generalised seizures without warning occurring during the daytime, are often reported with a frontal lobe focus, as spread is often rapid from that area.

▸▸ *pp 249-52*

4.9.2
EEG

- **Right anterior/fronto-temporal spike waves,** suggesting his epilepsy has a focal onset

4.9.3
Psychometric results:

- **Significant difference, suggesting an impairment in visuo-spatial abilities**
  - in a patient whose left hemisphere is dominant for language, this would suggest right hemisphere damage

PSYCHIATRIC HISTORY

At the age of 22, he developed episodes of paranoid ideation following clusters of seizures, where he would believe that colleagues were conspiring against him and talking about him in a derogatory way. He was admitted to hospital, was agitated and at times appeared paranoid and at times vacant. During one of these episodes, he attacked a nurse. These episodes of paranoid ideation tended to be self-limiting, remitting within days, usually without treatment.

At the age of 26, he had a cluster of tonic-clonic seizures, necessitating admission to a general medical hospital. After 2 days he experienced a pervading sense of unreality and became frightened and suspicious, with the belief that the nurses were injecting him with drugs to make him feel paranoid. He was then transferred to the care of the psychiatric services, where he was reported also to be experiencing visual hallucinations. On this occasion, the ideas of reference did not remit spontaneously, and he developed a depressed mood with suicidal ideation. He was treated with the antipsychotic medication risperidone. Over a period of several months there was some reduction in his paranoid ideation, and thus the neuroleptic medication was withdrawn. However, over the next year, he once again, developed the idea that his colleagues were talking about him and referring to him in a disparaging manner, which was accompanied by suicidal ideation. This did not follow an exacerbation of his seizures; in fact he had recently experienced a reduction in his seizure frequency. He was recommenced on risperidone and his paranoid thoughts improved. On antipsychotic medication, his psychotic ideation has remained in remission, and he has been able to return to work.

4.9.4

What psychiatric diagnosis would you consider?

(give two)

4.9.4

■ **Post ictal psychosis (PIP)**

His initial presentation would fit this category. Paranoid/ persecutory ideation is typical of the phenomenology of PIP. The episodes of psychosis experienced by this patient occurred after a cluster of seizures. This again is typical of PIP, when the seizure clusters are often precipitated by a reduction in anticonvulsant medication, either because of non-compliance or intentionally whilst being monitored as part of a pre-surgical assessment. Classically, episodes of PIP are self-limiting, patients returning to their pre-morbid mental state within a week, as in this case. However, if patients are very agitated/distressed, sedation may be helpful.

›› *pp 257-8*

■ **Chronic interictal psychosis**

(schizophrenia like psychosis of epilepsy, SLPE)

Although PIP can often be recurrent, with each episode having a similar phenomenology, progression to a chronic interictal psychosis (schizophrenia like psychosis of epilepsy, SLPE) has also been reported, often following a reduction in seizure frequency (as in this case). The clinical picture of SLPE is often of a paranoid psychosis, which may arise from a state of depersonalisation or derealisation. Hallucinations are usually auditory in nature, but visual hallucinations may occur and would be more suggestive of SLPE than schizophrenia. Negative symptoms are more unusual and affect tends to be well preserved.

Risk factors for the development of SLPE include:

Seizure type

- usually associated with brain damage
- complex partial commoner than primary generalised
- temporal lobe origin, especially spike foci in mediobasal area (left > right)
- onset of epilepsy before or around puberty, with onset of psychosis 10-14 years later
- often medically intractable
- 'forced normalisation' - EEG loses abnormal activity ('normalises')

Pathology

- 'Alien tissue lesions' (i.e. focal dysplasia, ganglioma or hamartoma) commoner than mesial temporal lobe sclerosis

Sex

- commoner in females

›› *pp 278-84*

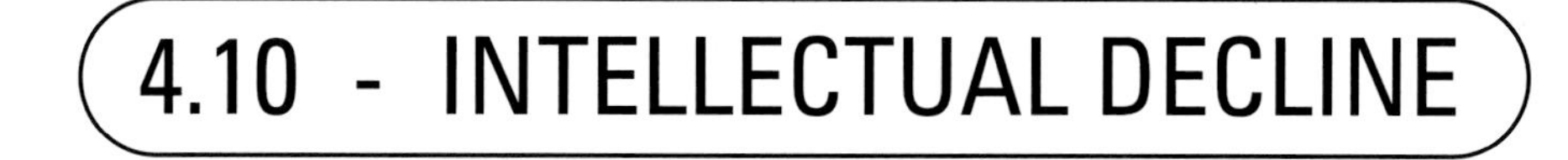

4.10 - INTELLECTUAL DECLINE

This section addresses the effect that epilepsy can have on cognitive function.

Cognitive function pp 260-5
See for reference

Exercise 4.10 VIGNETTE

A 34-year old man had no family history of epilepsy or psychiatric disorder. His birth and early development were normal, in particular he did not experience any febrile convulsions. He kept up with his classmates at school, although left without taking exams at the age of 16. He developed epilepsy at the age of 10. His first seizure occurred within an hour of waking and from the description was a generalised tonic clonic seizure, with no warning. He then experienced episodes of being vacant occurring several times a day. At the age of 15, he was referred to the neurology service after experiencing another generalised tonic clonic convulsion. An EEG showed widespread slow background activity (theta and delta waves) over both hemispheres. During sleep, spikes were recorded independently over both hemispheres. He was diagnosed as having primary generalised epilepsy – with both absence and tonic clonic seizures and he was started on sodium valproate. Despite high doses of valproate he continued to experience tonic-clonic seizures up to 15 times a month. On one occasion he sustained a fractured jaw during a seizure and on another he lacerated his scalp and needed sutures. At the age of 28, he assaulted his mother during a family argument and at the age of 30, he developed episodes during which he would be anxious, agitated, irritable, intimidating and disinhibited. His behaviour necessitated admission to psychiatric hospitals on several occasions and during one admission he threatened members of the nursing staff, necessitating his admission to a secure ward. Over the 20 years following the onset of his epilepsy, his family noticed a gradual deterioration in his memory. Neuropsychological assessments were performed and the results of the WAIS are shown below. He also performed badly in tasks assessing nonverbal recall and recognition memory. However, verbal learning was also significantly impaired. At the assessment performed when he was 34, there was also evidence of poor executive functioning.

4.10.1
What do you think his psychometric results (given below) suggest?

National Adult Reading Test (NART) IQ: 102
Age 28: Full Scale IQ: 84 (VIQ: 90; PIQ: 79)
Age 34: Full Scale IQ: 61 (VIQ: 69; PIQ: 57)

4.10.2
Describe the clinical features of epileptic dementia and list the causes of deterioration in IQ in people with epilepsy?
(highlight the factors that may be relevant in this case)

4.10.1
Psychometrics

- **Marked deterioration in his IQ**
  His NART IQ gives an indication of pre-morbid intelligence. There has been deterioration from baseline, at the time of testing when aged 28, and a further deterioration over the following 6 years.

- **Significant verbal-performance discrepancy**
- **Poor performance on non-verbal recall and recognition memory**
  Both suggest right hemisphere damage. The impairment of verbal learning, however, suggests bilateral temporal lobe involvement. The impairment of executive functioning implicates the pre-frontal cortex. Thus the wide range of deficits suggests global cerebral pathology.

4.10.2
Clinical features of Epileptic dementia

- **Decline in intellectual ability**
  Progressive impairment of memory, concentration and judgement
- **Severe personality deterioration**
- **Marked behaviour disorder**
  Impulsivity, irritability and outburtsts of rage
- **Neurotic and psychotic symptoms**

Epileptic dementia is a controversial and rare event, but can happen. Repeated fits can cause reactive gliosis and neuronal loss, especially in the hippocampus ('Sommers sector'), amygdala and dentate nucleus. Other vulnerable areas include the Purkinje cells in the cerebellum and pyramidal cells in the cortex. When intellectual function is impaired it generally reflects brain damage, but you should always suspect the anticonvulsant medication.

Factors relevant to this case:

- **recurrent head injuries**
- **epilepsy started in childhood**
- **frequent seizures**
- **valproate encephalopathy**
  may be a possibility in this case, following high doses of sodium valproate for many years. This is less frequently associated with cognitive decline than phenobarbitone (cognitive difficulties) or phenytoin (memory disorders). The more recent drugs are preferred but each individual may have an idiosyncratic response.

4.11 - RAGE & VIOLENCE

This concluding section takes two themes; offending behaviour and violence. In the last vignette in section 4.1.0, the patient exhibited episodes of violent behaviour (assaulting his mother and threatening nursing staff). It is often difficult in a patient with epilepsy to decide whether violent episodes are triggered by normal anger or 'episodic dyscontrol'. This section explores the issue in more detail.

»» ***Crime and epilepsy pp 273-5 & Disordered control of aggression pp 80-3***
See for further details

PLAY THE VIDEO

Exercise 4.11

Excerpt 4.11 features Dr Fenwick and Professor Goldberg discussing two subjects; how to assess offending behaviour in a person with epilepsy and how you might differentiate between violence stemming from epilepsy and 'normal' temper

4.11.1
What features would help you distinguish whether an offence or an episode of violence was related to epilepsy?

4.11.1

Criteria for establishing epilepsy as the cause for offending behaviour

- **Confirm diagnosis of epilepsy**
- **No planning**
- **Amnesia starting at time of seizure, not before**
- **Disorder of consciousness during index offence**
- **No attempt at concealment**

Violence secondary to epilepsy

- **Abrupt onset**
- **Non-directed and random**
- **Post-ictal confusion and amnesia of the event**
- **No guilt**

M4 SUMMARY

We've got to the end of module four.

The key learning points here has been to highlight the importance of identifying the types of seizure your patient has; differentiating other conditions to avoid unnecessary and inappropriate interventions and appreciating the related psychiatric associations.

MODULE 5 CONSULTANT ▸

Ian Everall

MODULE 5

Infection

CONTENTS

aims

This module aims to:
- introduce a range of the neuropsychiatric manifestations brought on by different cerebral infections
- highlight that cerebral infections account for both acute and chronic organic syndromes
- stress that a diverse range of infective agents (ie bacteria, parasites, fungi, and viruses etc) give rise to these clinical pictures depending on what country you're from

objectives

By the end of this module you should be able to:
- understand the variety of clinical pictures associated with HIV
- know the various causes and presentations of encephalitis and meningitis
- be aware that syphilis can mimic most neuropsychiatric conditions

PLAY THE VIDEO

Introduction 5.0

Excerpt 5.0 features Professor Everall with Professor Goldberg, discussing the assessment of a patient with a suspected cerebral infection.

Play the video and stop when prompted

pg 315-8

You may wish to read the introductory paragraph to Chapter 8 and the introduction to AIDS on pp 315-9 before starting section 5.1

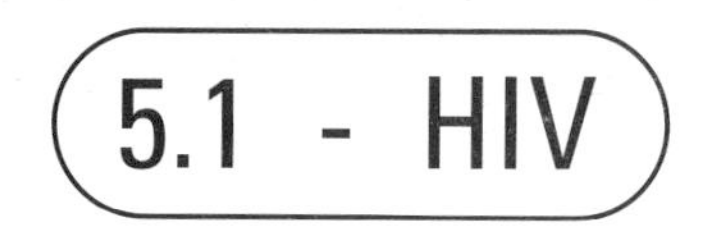

5.1 - HIV

There are a variety of clinical pictures associated with the Human Immunodeficiency Virus (HIV). This section starts with a clinical interview concerning a case of progressive cognitive impairment (HIV-associated dementia), the commonest central nervous system complication of HIV. The second part of section 5.1 uses a case vignette to lead you through other clinical pictures that may emerge.

▸▸ ***Classification of HIV-related diseases pp 318-33***
You may wish to refer to these pages for this next exercise

▶ PLAY THE VIDEO

Exercise 5.1

Excerpt 5.1 features Professor Everall interviewing a man whose partner suffers from HIV-related dementia.

Watch the video, then answer question 5.1.1

5.1.1
Name three key features of HIV dementia that are elicited?

Feedback is given over the page but try writing an answer before looking

FEED BACK

5.1.1

Three key features of HIV dementia elicited:

- **Cognitive abnormalities**
  - short-term memory difficulties (forgetfulness)
  - attention and concentration deficits
  - agnostic problems
    (e.g. understanding previously familiar objects)
- **Motor abnormalities**
  - incontinence
  - dressing dyspraxia
  - loss of fine motor control (e.g. difficulty holding cup)
  - inco-ordination
- **Behavioural change**
  - abusive
  - factuous and insightless (i.e. finding everything amusing, despite the gravity of the situation)
  - disinhibited
  - irritable
  - chaotic, with high risk behaviour (e.g. wandering)
  - deteriorated self-care

Pointers in the history that would suggest an opportunistic infection instead of HIV dementia:

- shorter duration
- more rapid progression
- pyrexia
- acute confusional state

⏩ ***HIV-associated dementia pp 324-6***

You may wish to study this topic in greater depth before moving onto the case vignette

Exercise 5.1 VIGNETTE

A 48-year-old man with known HIV infection, who does not attend for regular clinic checks, is brought to hospital as an emergency. He is confused, pyrexial, and unable to give a history as his speech is unintelligible. He is accompanied by a friend who informs you that over the last two to three months the patient has been getting increasingly forgetful, clumsy, and losing his balance. His behaviour has changed in that he can be rude to people and is spending a lot more money but appears unconcerned by the consequences of this. However, in the last two to three days the patient has become suddenly very confused, unable to dress himself properly or make any sense when he spoke.

On an initial clinical examination his cardiovascular and respiratory systems are unremarkable, there are no abdominal signs. Neurologically he is conscious, but appears disorientated. However it is difficult to assess him fully as he cannot comply with the examination, as he does not appear to understand what is being said to him. He is not on any medication and he has never taken anti-retroviral treatment.

5.1.2
What investigations would you perform?

⏩ ***pp 318-36***
You may wish to refer to these pages again whilst working through the vignette

5.1.2

You need to do a number of things –

- **Assess immune functioning and viral infection status**

  • **CD4 count**

  This tells you whether he is immunosuppressed and therefore vulnerable to opportunistic infections as well as disorders primarily due to HIV. If he is not immunosuppressed, then exclude an unrelated cerebral event.

  • **viral load test**

  This detects the number of RNA copies of the virus per ml of blood

- **Exclude systemic illness/infection or drug toxicity**

  You must ensure that these are not the cause of his confusional state.

  • **systemic illness/infection**

  Common systemic illnesses are pneumonia and gastrointestinal disorders, but patients can also suffer from urinary tract infections and septicaemia. Investigation of these will require a full blood count, urea and electrolytes, liver function tests, blood cultures, thick and thin blood films (if parasitic infections are suspected), chest X-ray, stool sample and urine sample. Syphilis serology should always be carried out.

  • **drug toxicity**

  Because of the limited nature of the history it is not clear whether this man is suffering from the toxic effects of drugs, whether prescribed or recreational. A drug screen would be valuable.

- **Further investigations of the central nervous system**

  • **neuroimaging e.g. MRI scan**

  An MRI scan of the head may reveal the presence of focal space occupying lesions, which are characteristic of opportunistic infections. Alternatively HIV itself can cause MRI brain changes. These include brain atrophy, which is more often ventricular than sulcal but both enlarged lateral ventricles and widened sulci can be observed. In addition, HIV can cause a diffuse hyperintensity of the cerebral white matter.

  • **lumbar puncture**

  Performed after the MRI scan has been carried out and raised intracranial pressure is excluded. The cerebrospinal fluid (CSF) is examined for cells, glucose, protein, and also antigens of known brain opportunistic infections. Also a viral RNA load can be performed on the CSF as an indication the amount of HIV in the brain compartment, as the higher this level is the more likely that HIV-related cognitive disorder (HIV-related dementia, HIV encephalitis) occurs.

The following results were obtained:

- chest X-ray, urea and electrolytes, haemoglobin, blood cultures, urine screen, liver function tests, and drug screen are all normal.
- peripheral white cell count and differential was normal
- syphilis serology was VDRL negative and FTA-antibody positive
- CD4 count is 55 which indicates severe immunosuppression *(normal range is 500-1,000 CD4 cells/ml blood)*
- viral Load is 250,000 RNA copies/ml.
  Current tests indicate that below 50 copies/ml is considered undetectable, while any level over 100,000 is considered high and associated with a poor prognosis
- MRI scan showed a focal mass of about 2cm diameter in the left fronto-temporal region
- lumbar puncture showed very high levels of cryptococcal antigen, and a high CSF viral RNA load of 600,000

5.1.3
What is the differential diagnosis?

5.1.4
Can you explain the unintelligible speech?

FEED BACK

5.1.3
Differential diagnosis

■ **AIDS (Acquired Immune Deficiency Syndrome)**
This man has evidence of severe immuosuppression, and with a CD4 count of below 200 cells/ml, in the absence of previous opportunistic infections, has a diagnosis of AIDS under CDC 1993 revision. Therefore he is vulnerable to both primary HIV pathology and secondary opportunistic infections. It is important to remember that more than one pathological process may be operating. The investigations have excluded systemic illness/pathology and drug toxicity as being aetiologically important. This indicates that the pathology is in the brain.

The history indicates that two events have occurred:

- **primary HIV-related brain disease**
  - due to high viral load in the CSF
  There was a longer history of cognitive decline (failing memory), motor abnormalities (clumsy and losing balance), and behavioural/personality change, which is typical of HIV-related cognitive impairment

- **secondary opportunistic infection in the brain**
  The recent history of acute confusion, unintelligible speech and pyrexia on examination tends to be more indicative of a secondary opportunistic infection. This is supported by identification of a focal lesion on MRI and the high cryptococcal antigen in the CSF. Cryptococcus neoformans is a mycosis (fungus) infection. Within the central nervous system infection typical results in a cryptococcal meningitis, but space occupying cryptococcomas can also occur.

■ **Syphilis**
The negative non-treponemal VDRL test together with a reactive treponemal test (FTA) is consistent with a past history of syphilis which was adequately treated. The non-treponemal tests are non-specific and yield false positives in a variety of acute and chronic conditions, such as viral illnesses, collagen vascular disease and pregnancy. The treponemal tests (FTA) are used to confirm a diagnosis of past or present infection; these tests usually remain positive for one year even after adequate treatment of syphilis.

▸▸ ***Syphilis pp 336-46***

5.1.4
Speech disorder

His unintelligible speech is either linked to the primary disorder or is secondary to his confusional state. It is difficult to assess this fully in such an ill patient. However, he seems to have difficulties in both comprehending speech and in expressive speech. The focal lesion may well affect Broca's area (inferior frontal gyrus) which can result in expressive dysphasia, and Wernicke's area (posterior portion of the superior temporal gyrus) which can produce a receptive aphasia.

On the assumption that the acute confusional state was caused by cryptococcus, the patient was started on intravenous amphotericin. Initially he kept removing the intravenous drip raising concern that the cryptococcal infection was not being adequately treated. Eventually he accepted the intravenous infusion and an adequate course of treatment was administered. There was, however, no improvement in his clinical state, and the focal lesion on MRI remained unchanged. Delayed microbiological results now showed that there were antibodies to toxoplasma gondii in the CSF and a further lumbar puncture revealed that the cryptococcal antigen was now negative.

5.1.5

What do you think is happening and what further treatment would you suggest ?

FEED BACK

5.1.5

The most likely explanation is that there are three pathologies in the brain of this patient.

- **Primary HIV infection**

  The HIV virus can cause a range of inflammatory disorders in the brain, neuronal damage (dendritic and synaptic loss), and neuronal death. The most well known inflammatory disorder is HIV encephalitis. The high level of virus in the brain, with ensuing inflammatory and neuronal damage, would expose the patient to the development of HIV associated dementia. The HIV infection, especially the high brain viral load will respond to combination antiretroviral therapy. This therapy usually consists of at least three antiretroviral agents. Some agents are better at brain penetration that others (especially, zidovudine, stavudine, and efavirenz). Not all the agents need to penetrate the brain as some improvement may be secondary to systemic reduction in viral load and consequent improvement of immune functioning, such as a rising CD4 count.

  The number of antiretroviral agents is constantly expanding and the reader is suggested to refer to any recent article on HIV treatment in order to become acquainted with current antiretroviral therapy practice.

  ▸▸ ***Primary HIV infection of the central nervous systempp 322-3***

- **Two Secondary opportunistic infections:**
  - **cryptococcal meningitis**
  - **toxoplasma gondii meningiencephalitis**

  The Cryptococcus is likely to have caused a cryptococcal meningitis which may have been difficult to elicit at the initial assessment. The negative CSF cryptococcal antigen indicates that this has been successfully treated with amphotericin. The assumption that the cryptococcus caused the focal lesion was probably wrong, and the lesion is more likely to have been a cyst in the brain caused by Toxoplasma gondii, a small protozoan infection. Toxoplasma is usually treated with sulphonamide and pyrimethamine.

  ▸▸ ***Opportunistic infections of the central nervous system pp 320-1***

  See also:

  ▸▸ ***Investigation and treatment pp 333-6***

  You may wish to read further details before moving onto section 5.2

5.2 - ENCEPHALITIS & MENINGITIS

Infections can effect either the meninges, giving meningitis with features of meningism, or the brain, leading to encephalitis, with features more consistent of acute or chronic confusional states. Encephalitis, in it's restricted sense, refers to a primary disease in which inflammation of the brain is caused by viral agents, although it can result from pyogenic infections or extensions of the inflamatory reaction in meningitis or cerebral absesses.

This section of the module starts with an exercise based around an excerpt of a man recovering from a cerebral infection. The latter part of section 5.2 deals with a case vignette which takes you through differential diagnosis and treatment issues.

▸▸ ***Encephalitis pp346-65 and Meningitis pp365-7***
You may wish to refer to these pages whilst tackling the exercises in this section

PLAY THE VIDEO

Exercise 5.2.1

Excerpt 5.2 features Professor David talking to a patient who describes an acute event five months prior to the recording, which has left him with some residual problems.

Watch the excerpt and then answer question 5.2.1. Feedback is given over the page but try answering the question before looking

5.2.1
List the abnormalities the patient describes and state what infection may have accounted for his presentation

FEEDBACK

5.2.1

Abnormalities described:

- **disorder of consciousness**
- **motor unsteadiness and weakness**
- **probable right hemianopia**
- **paraesthesiae**
- **epileptic seizures**
- **problems with time perception**
  (e.g. thinking he was in hospital for three days when he'd been in for five weeks)
- **extensive post-traumatic amnesia**
- **ongoing memory problems**
  (amnesia - telescoping events)

Δ **Herpes simplex encephalitis**

He describes a resolving acute organic syndrome and the persistance of a focal memory disturbance, which would point to herpes simplex encephalitis

⏩ *pp 356-8*

Exercise 5.2 VIGNETTE

Mr P is a 40-year-old professional who is brought to casualty after having been found wandering lost in his neighbourhood and talking unintelligibly. His wife says that although he is able to answer some direct questions he is becoming more detached from what is going on around him. She says that over the previous few weeks he has become more withdrawn, apathetic, and at times irritable. In the last few days he has also complained of headache, feeling nauseous and having a fever.

On examination it was difficult for Mr P to give sensible answers. His temperature was 37.9°C; there was a decrease in the level of consciousness and dysphasia, but evidence for both neck stiffness and photophobia were equivocal. There was no past medical history of note, and he is not taking any regular medication. Systemic causes of an organic dysfunction have been excluded. During the interview the wife recalled that three months ago that were on holiday in the Asian subcontinent when Mr P was bitten by a dog. Apart from thoroughly washing the bite, which appeared superficial, no further action was taken.

5.2.2 What is the differential diagnosis?
(give at least five)

5.2.3 List the main cause of viral encephalitis
(divide your answer into epidemic, sporadic and para-infectious causes)

5.2.4 List the main causes of meningitis
(give at least 3)

FEED BACK

5.2.2

Differential diagnosis

The most striking features are the recent behavioural change, headache, and impaired level of consciousness and pyrexia

Infective causes include:

- **Encephalitis**
  In the absence of any localising signs this is the most likely diagnosis. The prodromal illness and fever indicate an infectious cause of which viral encephalitis is common.
- **Meningitis or meningoencephalitis**
  Neck stiffness and photophobia would sugggest this, but the clinical findings were equivocal
- **Tuberculous meningitis**
- **Cerebral abscess**
  These can present with few definitive signs
  ⏩ *Cerebral abscess pg 368*

Other causes to exclude include:

- **Tumours**
- **Stroke**
- **Encephalopathy (e.g. hepatic)**

5.2.3

Viral causes of encephalitis

- **Epidemic virus infections**
  - enteroviruses
  - arthropod-borne viruses – e.g. tick borne encephalitis, Japanese B encephalitis, St Louis encephalitis
- **Sporadic virus infections**
  - herpes simplex virus types 1 and 2 (the commonest cause of sporadic encephalitis
  - herpes varicella-zoster - either as a post-infectious encephalitis after chicken pox, or as a complication of zoster reactivation
  - mumps virus – meningoencephalitis
  - rabies virus
- **Para-infectious**
  - influenza – as a post-infectious encephalitis
  - rubella virus – pan encephalitis as part of congenital rubella syndrome
  - measles virus – as either a post-infectious encephalitis or as subacute sclerosing panencephalitis

  ⏩ *Table 16 pg 347*

5.2.4

Main causes of meningitis

- **Bacterial** causes are principally due to meningococcus, Pneumococcus, Streptococcus, Staphylococcus, Haemophilus influenzae and Escherichia coli
- **Viral** causes result in an aseptic meningitis and include echoviruses, coxsackie virus group, mumps virus, Epstein Barr virus, and human immunodeficiency virus
- **Tuberculous meningitis** – which often has an insidious onset with low grade pyrexia, often slight neck stiffness and can be difficult to diagnose
- **Fungal -** cryptococcus

  ⏩ *Meningitis pp 365-8*

Mr P is admitted to hospital and a CT brain scan shows focal areas of low attenuation in both temporal lobes with areas of haemorrhage. An EEG shows periodic spike and slow wave activity over both temporal lobes. A lumbar puncture reveals a blood stained cerebrospinal fluid (CSF) with the following results:

CSF results

- 900 blood cells $\times 10^6$/l
- 43 white cells $\times 10^9$/l, 60% lymphocytes
- Sugar 3.6mmol/l (blood sugar 5.0)
- Protein 1.6g/l
- No organisms seen

5.2.5 What is the diagnosis?

5.2.6 What other investigations can be performed and describe the results you may expect?

5.2.7 What is the treatment for this condition?

5.2.8 Should attention still be paid to the dog bite?

5.2.5

Diagnosis

- **Herpes simplex encephalitis**
  The bloody CSF is compatible as the presence of red cells reflects haemorrhagic necrosis
  ›› *pp 356-7*

5.2.6

Expected results:

- **Paired samples of CSF/blood**
  May show serial rising titres of viral antigens. A CSF sample may also show lymphocytes, leucocytosis and raised protein and normal glucose.
- **Polymerase chain reaction for viral DNA**
  Provides a rapid virological test result on samples of CSF
- **Brain biopsy**
  Tissue will show areas of haemorrhage and necrosis, neuronal death, lymphocytic cuffing of vessels, and astrocyte proliferation. Eosinophilic Type A inclusion bodies may be observed in the surviving neurones. The presence of Herpes simplex can be confirmed immuno-cytochemically to detect herpes virus antigen.
- **EEG**
  Typical appearance of periodic spike and slow wave activity in temporal lobes
- **Neuroimaging**
  Low density areas on CT in the temporal lobes

5.2.7

Treatment

Intravenous acyclovir for a minimum of 10 days.

5.2.8

Dog bite - importance of Rabies

Rabies gives a non-specific prodrome lasting two to seven days, which can include fever and severe malaise. Behavioural disturbances occur, including hyperactivity, insomnia, hallucinations, anxiety and aggressive behaviour. In about 50% of cases, abnormal sensation at the bite site is reported. An incubation of up to one year follows – at this point the history of a bite or observing the telltale scar is critical. The onset of illness is then sudden with pyrexia, excitement, hydrophobia and violent muscular spasms (particulary of the oesophagus and respiratory muscles).

Two clinical forms are described:

'Furious' rabies (more common), characterised by hyperexcitability, spasms and hydrophobia

'Dumb' rabies – presents with an ascending paralysis

Bites from rabid animals do not always result in disease. Factors that may influence this process include the severity of the bite (determines the viral dose) and the site of the bite, with head and neck carrying the greatest risk. Despite best efforts, including modern intensive care, antiviral and immunomodulatory drugs, the disease is invariably fatal

›› *pg 359*

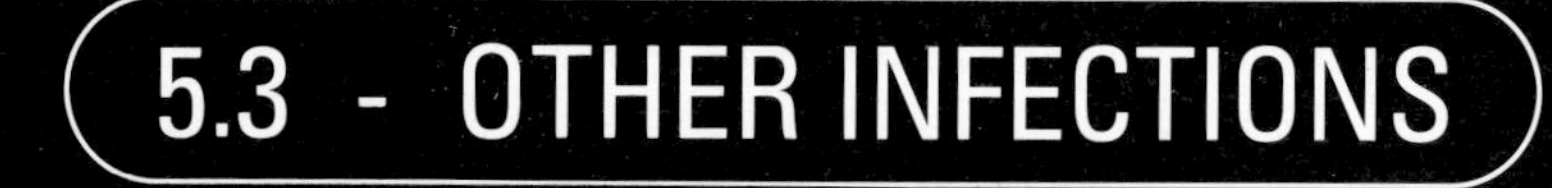

5.3 - OTHER INFECTIONS

This final section of the module uses scans taken from a range of other cerebral infections. The aim is to highlight some neuroimaging findings that characterise these infections.

> ▸▸ ***Other infective processes pp 368-74***
> *You may wish to refer to these pages whilst thinking of conditions that may have contributed to the findings in scans 5.3.1 - 5.3.3*

Exercise 5.3

Describe any abnormalities you can see on each scan and suggest a likely diagnosis

Feedback is given after the scans but try answering each question before looking

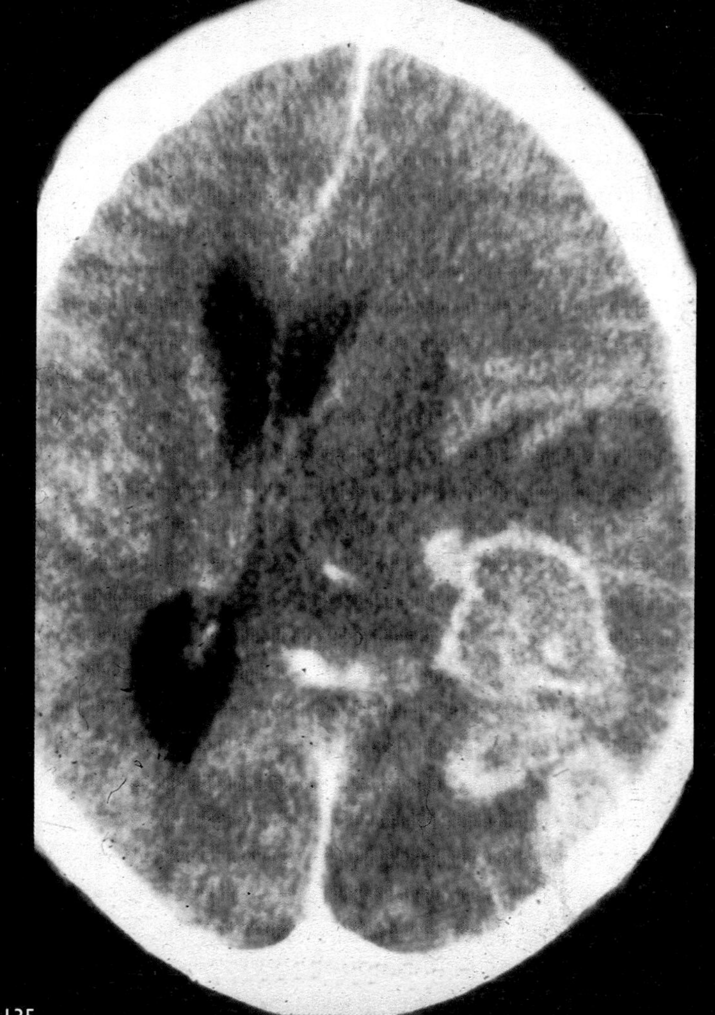

5.3.1

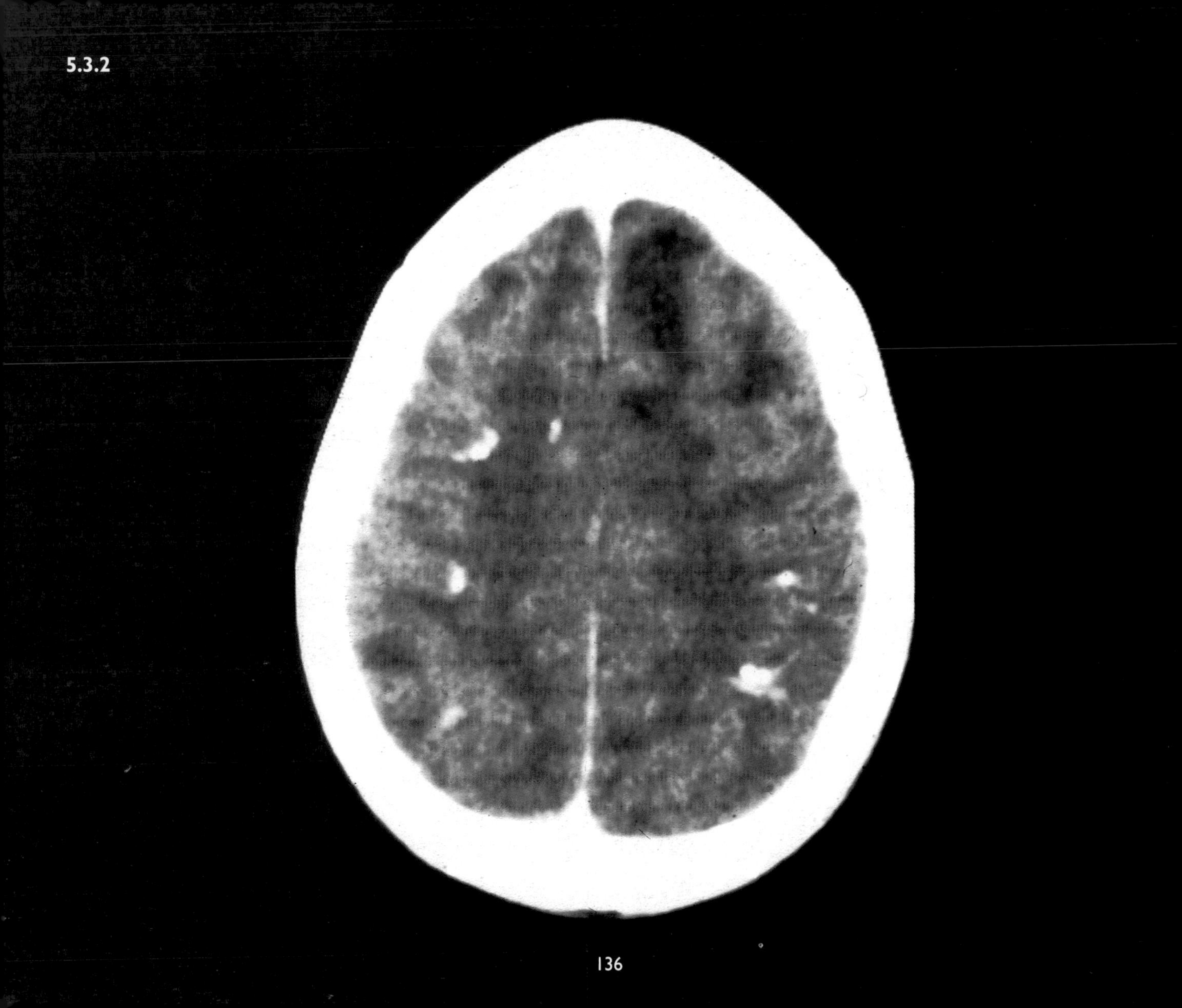
5.3.2

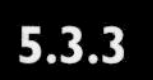
5.3.3

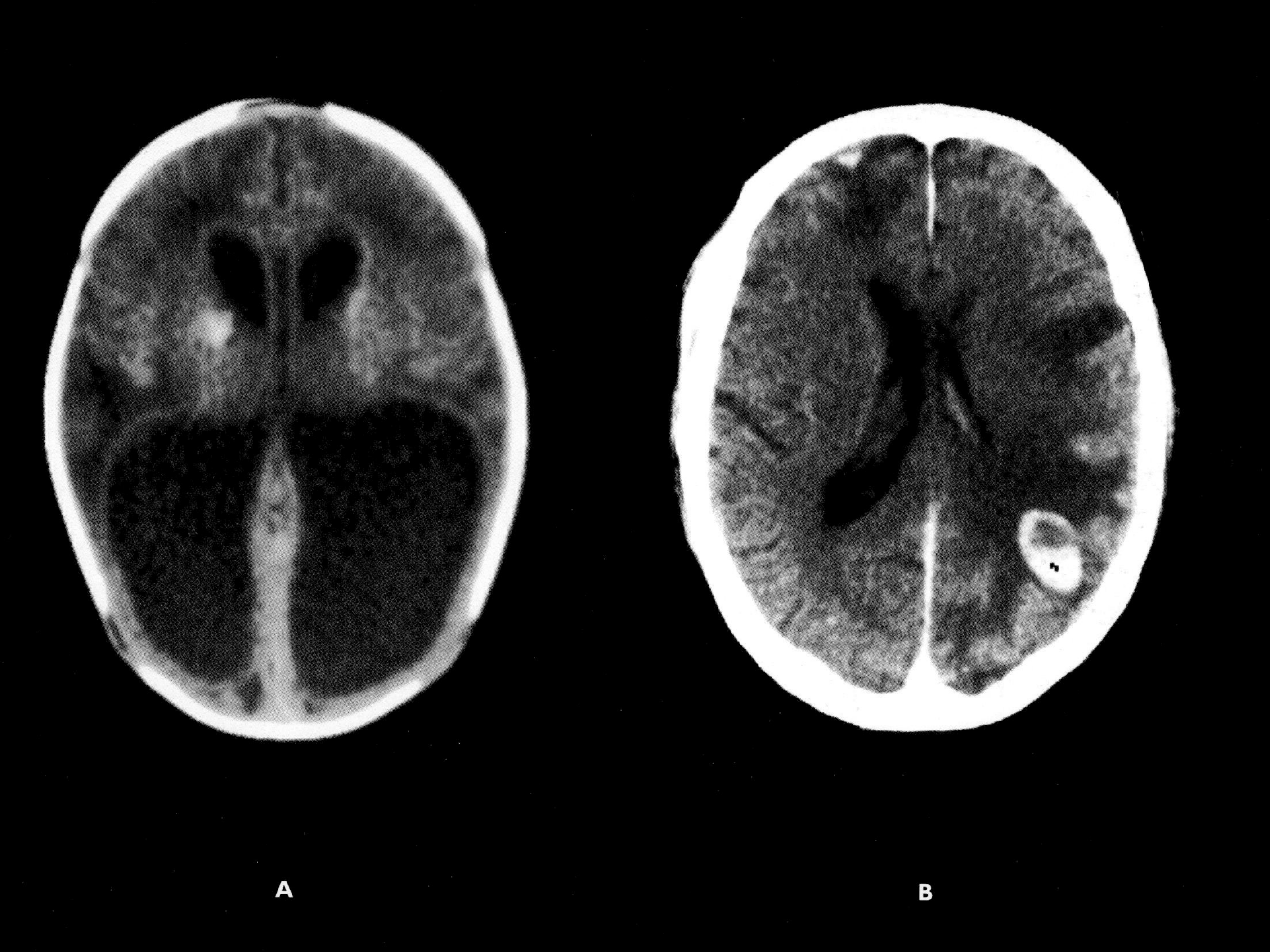

5.3.1

- **Tuberculoma**

The image is a CT scan with contrast, showing multiple, loculated thick walled structures in the left tempero-occipital lobe with a large mass effect.

(ΔΔ tumour, abscess and granulomas e.g. ⏩ ***Sarcoid pp 763-5***)

5.3.2

- **Cysticercosis**

The image is a CT scan showing calcification (white spots) at the border of the grey/white intersection. The size and proportion of these spots are fairly characteristic of Cysticercosis. ⏩***pg 370***

5.3.3

- **Congenital Toxoplasmosis (Scan A)**

CT scan (with no contrast) of the posterior frontal and mid-parietal lobes of a neonate showing a combination of delayed development, with localised ependymal disease.

Abnormalities shown include:

- widening of the posterior ventricles and virtually no parietal lobe tissue
- widening of the anterior horns
- low attenuation of the frontal white matter
- high attenuation of the ventricular ependyma (indicating ependymitis), including a localised right frontal 'abscess'
- general cortical atrophy

Other, less likely, causes include bacterial or viral infections (e.g. TB or AIDS) and Tuberous Sclerosis

- **Acquired Toxoplasmosis (Scan B)**

CT scan post contrast - (note falx is easily seen) - of a young man with AIDS and secondary Toxoplasmosis.

Abnormalities include

- enhancing lesions: left parietal, right frontal convexity and very small nodules on the right grey/white matter junction
- low attenuation related to the two larger lesions (i.e. oedema)
- mass effect in the left posterior horn

ΔΔ absesses, neoplasia (secondary deposits), emboli or inflammation (e.g. subacute bacterial encephalitis)

See also:

⏩ ***Other infections pp 368-74***

- *Lyme disease*
- *Typhus*
- *Trypanosomiasis*
- *Malaria*
- *Chronic fatique disorder*
- *Rheumatic fever*

M5 SUMMARY

We've got to the end of module five.

There are several key elements here; the aetiology is multiple but that the clinical picture is of both acute and chronic organic reactions (with features secondary to encephalitis, meningitis or space occupying lesions).

Brian Toone

MODULE 6

Dementia

CONTENTS

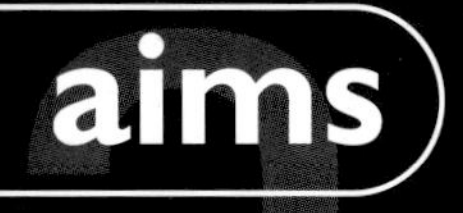

objectives

This module aims to:

- review the disorders which give rise to progressive cognitive impairment and personality change
- contrast an approach of looking at dementias from a neuropathological and a syndromal perspective
- highlight key cognitive abnormalities that accompany dementia syndromes

At the end of this module you should be able to:

- have an understanding of the disease processes which cause dementia
- be familiar with the neuropathology of the commoner causes of dementia
- be familiar with the mode of presentation, course and prognosis of the principle dementia syndromes

PLAY THE VIDEO

Introduction 6.0

Excerpt 6.0 features Dr Toone with Professor Goldberg, discussing an outline of how to go about assessing someone you might suspect has a dementia syndrome.

Play the video and stop when prompted

pp 428-9
You may wish to read the introductory paragraphs to Chapter 10 before starting section 6.1

6.1 - NEUROPATHOLOGY

This section looks at dementia from a neuropathological perspective using a series of neuroimages showing cerebral changes associated with different dementing processes. Different neuropathologies have predilections for certain areas but it's not easy to predict the eventual neuropathology on the basis of the clinical presentation and course (Alzheimer's and multi-infarct dementia are easier than frontotemporal dementia). Structural and functional neuroimaging are facilitating differentaition during life, but often it is not until post-mortem that the true pathology is reavealed.

▸▸ ***pp 495-7 Investigations***

You may wish to read further details on this topic before tackling this exercise

Exercise 6.1

This exercise features four different conditions covered by the scans 6.1.1-6.1.4.

For each scan, write an answer to the question below

What abnormalities can you see and what possible diagnosis might account for these changes?

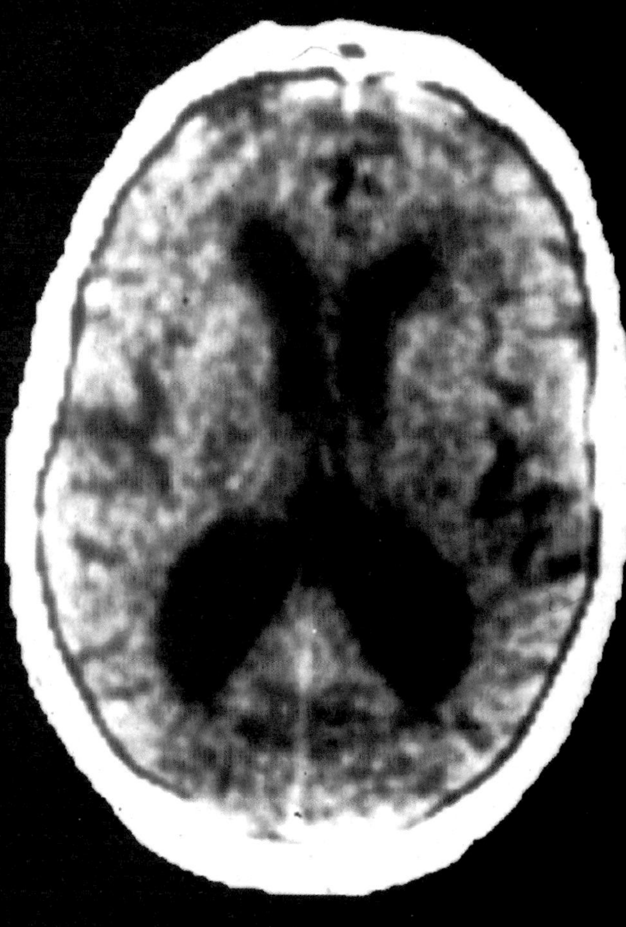

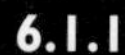

6.1.1

6.1.2

6.1.3

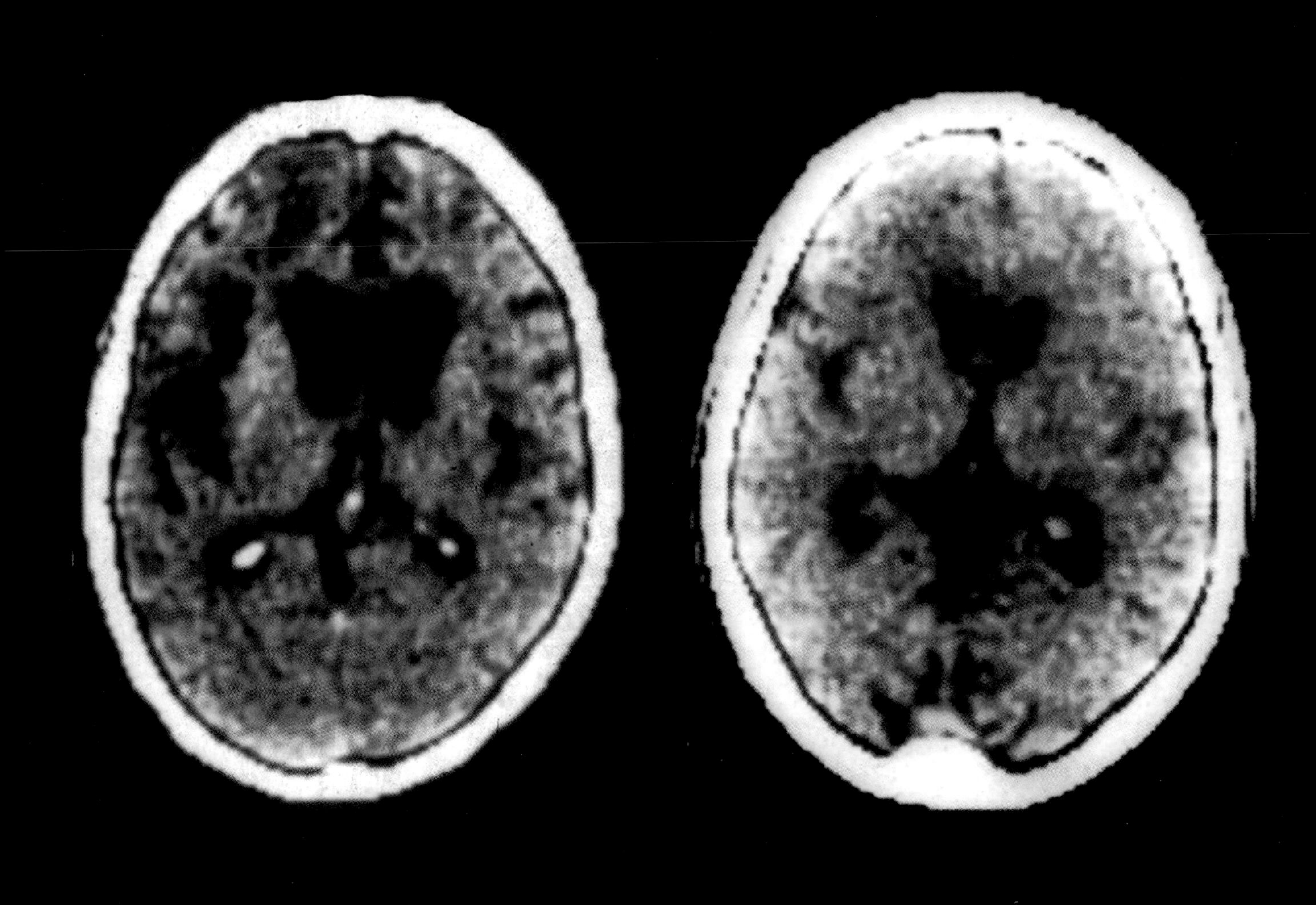

6.1.4

Scan A and B are of the same patient

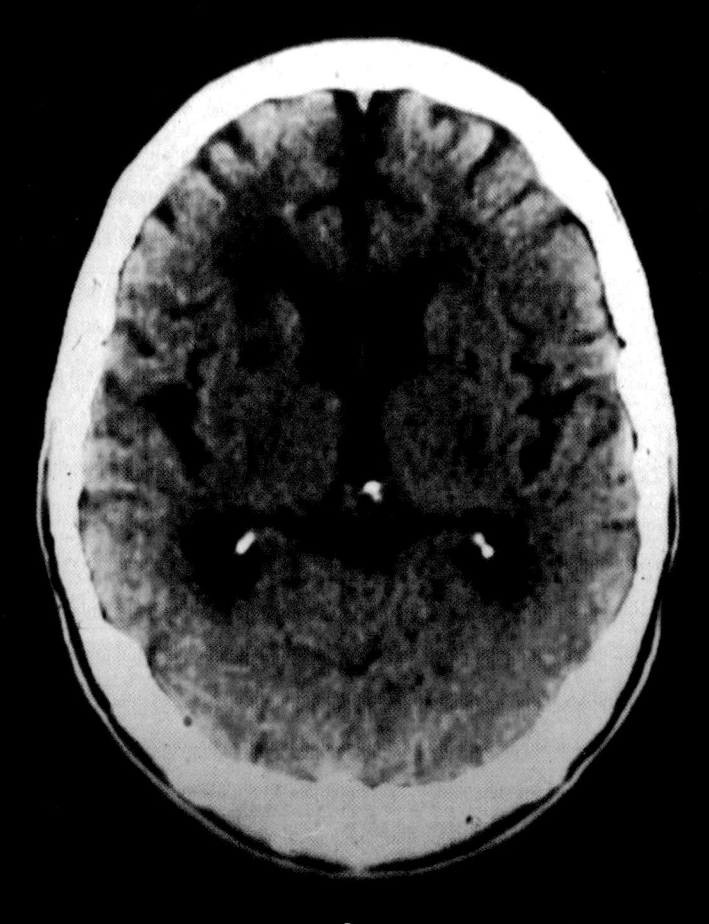

A

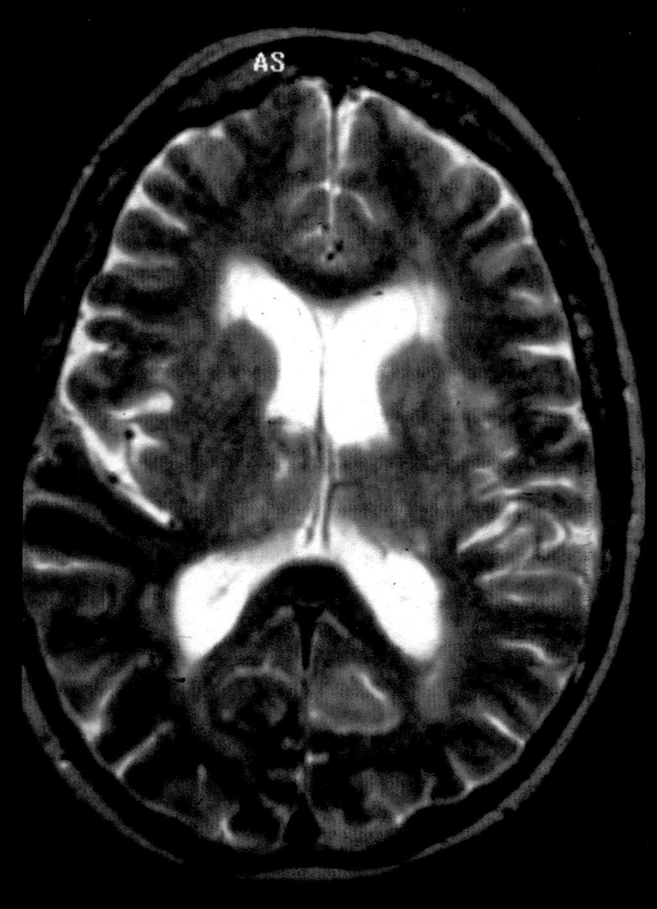

B

FEED BACK

6.1.1

■ **Advanced Alzheimer's disease**

Transverse CT scan showing symetrical enlargement of Sylvian fissures and choroidal fissures reflecting a grossly atrophied brain. The cortical atrophy tends to affect the frontotemporal lobes more severely than the parieto-occipital regions. You would need a coronal view to demonstrate temporal atrophy (seen in module 2).

- ***Alzheimer's disease pp 437-50***
- ***Plate 10 Senile (neuritic) plaque pg xx***

6.1.2

■ **Pick's disease**

CT scan showing asymmetrical cerebral atrophy (right > left) confined to the anterior half of the brain. The diagnosis was confirmed at autopsy; making the diagnosis during life is very difficult unless there is a strong familial component.

- ***Pick's disease pp 460-3***

6.1.3

■ **Huntington's disease**

The heads of the caudate are atrophic, shown by lack of the normal convex bulging into the lateral walls of the frontal horns of the lateral ventricles (this is characteristic). There is little by way of sulcal enlargement; the damage is sub-cortical.

- ***Huntington's disease pp 465-73***
- ***plate 19 on pg xxiii***

6.1.4

■ **Arteriopathic - Binswanger's disease**

CT (scan A) and MRI T2 axial (scan B) showing ventricular dilatation accompanied by enlargement of cortical sulci and Sylvian fissures. The anterior horns of the lateral ventricles are 'capped' by areas of white matter translucency on MRI T2 ('leukoaraiosis'). They appear darker on the CT and correspond to increased fluid. Small subcortical infarcts are apparent in the heads of the caudate nuclei and right thalamus (on MRI)

- ***Subcortical arteriosclerotic encephalopathy pp 458-60***
- ***Multi-infarct dementia pp 453-8***
- ***Dementia as a sequelae of stroke pp 383-4***

For further discussion on neuropathology:

- ***Senile dementia of Alzheimer type pp 429-37***
- ***Lewy body dementia pp 450-3***
- ***Lewy bodies in the substantia nigra plate 11/12 pg xxi***
- ***Frontal lobe dementia pp 463-5***
- ***Creutzfeldt-Jakob disease pp 473-9 + plate 16 pg xxii***
- ***Alcohol dementia pp 603-7***
- ***Other disorders producing dementia pp 751-62***

6.2 - DIFFERENTIAL DIAGNOSIS

Differentiating dementia syndromes, as opposed to neuropathology, is an alternative approach to understanding dementia. Consideration is given to phenomenology in relation to areas of diseased brain rather than specific neuropathology. The remainder of this module uses a series of clinical interviews to address the clinical presentations of the dementia syndrome. The key point to bear in mind is the immense variability of presentations of dementia, making accurate diagnosis during life extremely difficult. Two main threads determine the clinical picture; the aetiological nature of the condition and the part of the brain damaged (including secondary spread). These don't necessarily run in parallel.

The exercise in this section explores these difficulties.

▸▸ ***Assessment and differential diagnosis pp 490-7***
Consult this reference if you get stuck

▶ PLAY THE VIDEO

Exercise 6.2

Excerpt 6.2 features Dr Toone interviewing a woman and her husband, highlighting some difficulties brought on by dementia. The excerpt starts with how her problems began, and then goes on to highlight some of the difficulties she subsequently started to notice.

Watch excerpt 6.2, then answer questions 6.2.1- 6.2.2
You'll find feedback over the page but try writing something down before checking the answers.

6.2.1
What cognitive abnormalities does she describe that suggest an organic impairment?
(give at least two)

6.2.2
What is your differential diagnosis ?
(we suggest three)

6.2.1
Cognitive abnormalities featured include:

- **Performance decline**
  Heralding the onset of her difficulties (an error at work), followed by an increasing struggle with organisational tasks.

- **Topographical disorientation**
  (indicating a probable bilateral posterior parietal lesion)
  She also describes a catastrophic reaction when she realises that she can no longer make sense of a map whilst orientering *(which is a race between points, requiring linking a map with landmarks to find your route)*. She then describes experiencing difficulty finding her way around familiar surroundings (i.e. the local streets of her home town)

- **Concentration and attention deficits**
- **Memory failure**

  Difficulty registering new events, with the result that she repeats the same things over and over (a perseverative tendency that she exhibits on the excerpt)

6.2.2
ΔΔ

- **Alzheimer's**
  In this woman's case, early topographical disorientation and a disproportionate degree of spatial disorientation has set in which is normally a late phenomenon. Memory is usually the first cognitive function ravished by this illness.
  ⏩ ***Alzheimer's disease pp 437-50***

- **Multi infarct dementia**
  (affecting right parietal lobe)
  ⏩ ***Multi infarct dementia pp 453-8***

- **Pseudodementia**
  Note how in this woman's case, she had a history of unipolar affective disorder and for some time her symptoms had been misdiagnosed as depressive, illustrating how difficult it can be in clinical practice to make the distinction. Note how she could subjectively distinguish the cognitive dysfunction experienced in depression compared with dysfunctions at the onset of her dementia.
  ⏩ ***Depressive pseudodementia pp 485-90***

See also
⏩ ***Pseudodementias pp 479-85 and 489-90***
⏩ ***Dementia questionnaires and rating scales pp122-6***

6.3 - FOCAL DEMENTIA SYNDROMES

The exercise in this section looks at the situation where a patient presents with a relatively discrete, focal dementia syndrome. The questions test your observational ability and encourage you to consider different options that may account for the difficulties described and demontrated.

PLAY THE VIDEO

Exercise 6.3

Excerpt 6.3 features an interview between Dr Toone, a patient and her husband. It starts with a description of the onset of the disorder and concludes with selected aspects of the cognitive examination.

Watch the excerpt and then try the questions below. Feedback is given over the page but try answering each question before looking.

6.3.1
List the functions that are principally affected and those that are spared?
(give at least three)

6.3.2
What do you think is the diagnosis and the site of her brain lesion?

6.3.3
What other possible diagnoses are there?
(Give at least five and for each possible diagnosis noting any features that would make the diagnosis unlikely)

FEED BACK

6.3.1

Functions affected:

- **Semantic component of language and memory**
  Her ability to understand the meaning of many words and objects is severely impaired - "what's recognise?" Her problems go beyond an inability to name objects - she cannot describe them, or say what they are for (e.g. telephone). She retains some vague knowledge of the use of objects, e.g. holding the phone to her ear and using the comb and stapler.
- **Proposagnosia** - she can't recognise her work colleagues
- **Colour anomia** - she finds difficulty naming colours
- **General memory impairment**

Functions spared:

- **Visuo-spatial abilities** - still being able to find her way around, using maps
- **Non-verbal memory** - remembers tunes but not words
- **Motor functions** - shows no signs of dyspraxia, retaining the ability to dance and drive a car
- **Insight**

6.3.2

- **Diagnosis: Semantic dementia**
  In semantc dementia there is a dense loss of semantic knowledge, starting with problems of language comprehension (loss of semantic encoding - i.e. visual and verbal objects lose their meanig). Verbal fluency is impaired, reflecting an impoverished vocabulary. It can be difficult to tease out a primary semantic dementia, from primary progressive dysphasia.
- **Lesion - Dominant temporal lobe**
  Loss of semantic information has been associated with damage to the anterior temporal cortex, although no definitive neuropathology has been identified. Fronto-temporal dementias tend to be asymmetrical and marked if affecting the dominant hemisphere.The clinical presentation depends on which part of the brain is affected at onset, and which systems are damaged by spread.

▸▸ ***Semantic dementia pp 753-4***

6.3.3

Other diagnosis:

- **Primary progressive aphasia** - illness also starts with word finding difficulties, but proceeds to dysphasias and dyspraxias. Patients may become mute and focal neurological signs may be manifest. The patient in this excerpt retains social skills and the ability to drive, so this diagnosis would be less likely.

  ▸▸ ***Primary progressive aphasia pp 752-3***
- **Frontal lobe dementia -** but personality changes are not marked
- **Alzheimer's (early)** - unlikely given the preservation of other functions
- **Pick's disease** - but speech prodution appears spared
- **Diencephalic tumour** - marked amnesic features occur and confabulation are common

  ▸▸ ***Diencephalic tumour pp 227-9***

6.4 - OTHER DEMENTIA SYNDROMES

The final section of this module presents an example of a case of dementia brought on by more generalised neuropathology

PLAY THE VIDEO

Exercise 6.4

Excerpt 6.4 features Dr Lovestone interviewing a patient. The patient is orientated in person and place. The interview starts with further questions that feature in the Mini-mental state examination (▸▸ ***pg 123***) and concludes with a description of some unusual phenomena.

Watch the video, then answer questions 6.4.1-6.4.3. Feedback is given over the page but try answering each question before looking

6.4.1
Which diagnosis is strongly suggested, and how common is it?
(give the diagnostic features of this disease)

6.4.2
What is the practical importance of this diagnosis?

6.4.3
Are investigations usually helpful?
(If so, which ones?)

6.4.1

- **Lewy body dementia**
  Strongly suggested by description of visual and auditory hallucinations. Lewy body dementia is now regarded as perhaps the second commonest cause of dementia - 20% of all cases

  ▸▸pp 450-3

Distinguishing features (not described):

- extra-pyramidal signs; parkinsonism
- temporal variability of symptoms (similar to vascular dementia)
- fluctuating course
- late onset with a rapid progression

NOTE

The dementia in Parkinson's also has Lewy bodies in the substantial nigra and cortex, but unlike Lewy body dementia, there would be a long history of parkinson symptoms.

6.4.2

- **Intolerance to antipsychotics**
  Patints with Lewy body disease have an intolerance to antipsychotics and anticholinergics. There would be a severe adverse reaction if these visual hallucinations were treated with neuroleptics.

6.4.3

Investigations are usually unhelpful in this condition, although the following may point towards the diagnosis:

- **CSF showing possible elevated protein**
- **EEG showing diffuse slowing**
- **Neuroimaging showing diffuse atrophy**

See also

▸▸ Management of the senile and presenile dementias pp 497-506

M6 SUMMARY

We've got to the end of module six.

The module contrasted the neuropathology of dementia with the clinical syndromes, stressing that aetiological factors are multiple and the clinical picture will be governed by what areas of the brain are most affected.

K Ray Chaudhuri

MODULE 7

Movement disorders

CONTENTS

aims

This module aims to:

- highlight the presentation and problems associated with parkinsonism
- demonstrate the striking clinical picture of Tourette's syndrome
- present a series of different clinical manifestations of movement disorders

objectives

By the end of the module you should be able to:

- describe the physical manifestations of movement disorders
- outline the subcortical neuropathology implicated in these abnormal movements
- understand the neuropsychiatric conditions associated with the different disorders

PLAY THE VIDEO

Introduction 7.0

Excerpt 7.0 features Dr Chaudhuri and Professor Goldberg, discussing important issues in the history and examination of someone suspected of having a movement disorder

Play the video and stop when prompted

pg 639

You may wish to read the introductory three paragraphs to Chapter 14 before starting section 7.1

7.1 - PARKINSONISM

We start with a look at a condition that highlights the interplay between subcortical dysfunction and neuropsychiatric disorders. Parkinson's disease, characterised by subcortical neuronal loss and Lewy body formation, is associated with an increased incidence of both depression and dementia. The parkinsonian syndrome - tremor, rigidity and abnormal movements (bradykinesis and postural anomalies) - is a broader concept, having several aetiological causes and neuropsychiatric associations.

The aim of the exercise in this section is to show a clinical interview of a patient who describes features of parkinsonism, and displays several movement disorders. The questions posed test your observational powers and knowledge of treatments available.

▸▸ ***Parkinson's disease and the parkinsonian syndrome pp 646-52***

You may wish to read up about the clinical features, differential diagnosis and treatment before tackling the exercise

▶ PLAY THE VIDEO

Exercise 7.1

Excerpt 7.1 features Dr Chaudhuri interviewing a man presenting with a ten year history of Parkinson's disease.

NOTE

The drug 'sinemet' is mentioned in the interview; the generic name is co-careldopa (a mixture of carbidopa and levodopa)

Watch the video, then answer questions 7.1.1. - 7.1.5. You'll find feedback over the page, along with further reading, but try writing something down before checking the answers.

7.1.1 What abnormal involuntary movements are visible during the interview and what are they due to?
(give at least 3)

7.1.2 What are the differential diagnoses?
(give at least three)

7.1.3 What is apomorphine and how is it useful in movement disorders?

7.1.4 What other disturbances (besides movement disorders) are evident during the interview?
(give at least 3)

7.1.5 What could be the reason for postural dizziness?

FEED BACK

7.1.1

Abnormal involuntary movements visible during the interview:

- **Generalised chorea/dystonia** (e.g. left hand and ankle)
- **Craniocervical dystonia** (right rotational torticollis)
- **Akathisia**

These are levodopa induced dyskinesias and result from long term dopaminergic therapy. The levodopa syndrome is characterised by 'wearing off' (end-dose deterioration) and 'on-off' fluctuations. The current movements are secondary to another feature of the syndrome; 'peak dose' chorea and akathisia while the patient is 'on'. The patient also describes the parkinsonian features of resting hand tremor, rigidity (stiffness) and bradykinesia with akinesia (freezing)

»***pp 650-1*** *for further discussion*

7.1.2

This man suffers from early young onset Parkinson's disease but the differential diagnoses could include:

- **Drug induced parkinsonism** »***pp 640***
- **Dopa responsive dystonia** (Segawa's disease) »***pp 671***
- **Wilson's disease** »***pp 661-6***
- **Huntington's chorea** »***pp 465-73***
- **Striatonigral degeneration** »***pp 668-9***

7.1.3

Apomorphine

- **An injectable potent D1 and D2 dopamine receptor agonist**

  Apomorphine is used in advanced Parkinson's disease with motor response fluctuations due to 'on-off' periods and is effective because its subcutaneous route via a pump every 12, 18 or 24 hrs, gives a rapid onset of action

» ***pp 651***

7.1.4

Other disturbances of Parkinson's disease evident during the interview are:

- **Non-motor complications**
  - sleep disturbance
  - dysarthria (mild)
  - sweating problems
- **Neuropsychiatric problems**
  - depression/mood swings/aggression/forgetfulness

» ***'Psychiatric aspects of Parkinsonism' pp 652-61***

7.1.5

Postural dizziness:

- **Iatrogenic postural hypotension**
- **Autonomic Failure**

» ***Progressive supranuclear palsy and Corticobasal degeneration pp 666-8***

You may also wish to read about for further details on other subcortical disorders with neuropsychiatric sequelae

7.2 - TOURETTE'S SYNDROME

Tourette's syndrome is an example of a disorder where it's difficult to establish exactly what influence mental processes have on the motor dysfunctions observed. The exercise in this section aims to demonstrate the striking features of this disorder and test your knowledge of the treatment options.

▸▸ ***Gilles de la Tourette's syndrome pp 680-7***
You may wish to read up about the clinical features, differential diagnosis and treatment before tackling the exercise

▶ P L A Y T H E V I D E O

Exercise 7.2

Excerpt 7.2 features Professor Robertson with a mother and her son who shows a particularly severe form of the disorder.

Watch excerpt 7.2, then answer questions 7.2.1- 7.2.3. You'll find feedback over the page but try writing something down before checking the answers.

7.2.1
What classical features of Tourette's syndrome are shown or described?
(list at least 5)

7.2.2
What other features are not shown (described)?
(list at least 2)

7.2.3
What treatments can help this condition?
(list 2, giving examples of each)

FEEDBACK

7.2.1

Features shown:

- **Multiple motor tics**
  Simple and complex tics of the face, head, trunk and limbs
- **Compulsions to hit and punch his own body**
- **Occasional complex co-ordinated movements**
  e.g. placing hands on mother's shoulders
- **Vocalisations** - grunts and barks
- **Coprolalia** - rude utterances
- **Copropraxia** - rude gestures

Features described:

- **Onset in childhood**
- **Resultant impairment in social functioning**

NOTE

- *Agrophobia and depression, with suicidal ideation*
- *Adverse effect on family e.g. aggravating mother's panic attacks*

7.2.2

Other features (not shown/described):

- Echolalia
- Echopraxia
- Obsessive compulsive disorder

7.2.3

Treatments:

- Behavioural therapy
  - Operant conditioning
- Pharmacotherapy
  - Haloperidol
  - Pimozide
  - Sulpiride
  - Clonadine

▸▸ ***Gilles de la Tourette's syndrome pp 680-7***

If you need to consolidate the points raised in this section you may wish to re-read and then replay the excerpt

7.3 - DIFFERENTIAL DIAGNOSIS

This section concludes the module with a series of excerpts of different clinical presentations. The aim here is to test your ability to identify clinical signs and link these findings with the disorders they highlight.

- ***Drug-induced disorders pp 639-46***
- ***The dystonias pp 669-80***

You may wish to read further details before tackling the exercise

PLAY THE VIDEO

Exercise 7.3

Excerpts 7.3.1 - 7.3.7 feature brief glimpses of motor dysfunctions

Watch each excerpt separately. For each, write down an answer to question below. Look at the feedback over the page after you've watched the whole series and written an answer for each excerpt.

What abnormal motor movements are being shown ?

7.3.1 Young woman with contorted facial expression

7.3.2 Man holding out his hands and trying to hold a glass of water

7.3.3 Man who has been asked to turn around

7.3.4 Woman sticking her tongue out

7.3.5 Woman's face, close up

7.3.6 Woman chanting, dressed as a nun

7.3.7 Man leaning over

7.3.1

- **Acute dystonia**
  Abnormal muscle tone (especially head and neck), leading to facial spasm and a severe, fixed upward gaze. This may persist for hours if untreated with anticholinergics (e.g. procyclidine)

  ➧ *Acute dystonia pg 641 and pg 644*

7.3.2

- **Benign essential tremor**
  Bilateral distal, and proximal, postural and kinetic tremor with reduction at rest

  ➧ *Differential diagnosis pg 649*

7.3.3

Advanced Parkinson's disease with:

- **Shuffling gait**
- **Turning difficulty**
- **Freezing** (akinesia)
- **Finger and Body bradykinesia**
- **Facial impassivity**

  ➧ *Parkinsonism pg 640*

7.3.4

- **Oro-facio-lingual dyskinesias**
  Spectrum of drug induced tardive dyskinesias; purposeless, repetitive hyperkinesias, especially of the mouth, tongue and jaw. The patient has some degree of voluntary suppression and the motor dysfunction disappears in sleep

  ➧ *Tardive dyskinesia pp 641-2*

7.3.5

- **Blepharospasm or Left hemifacial spasm**
  Uncontrollable tendency to spontaneous and forcible eye closure - shown in the excerpt as spasm of the orbicularis oculi

  ➧ *Blepharospasm pp 678-9*

7.3.6

- **Akathisia**
  Akathisia is the subjective experience of restlessness, often accompanied by incessant movement. The patient is unable to sit or stand still - as shown in the excerpt. The presentation also highlights how this condition may often get misdiagnosed as psychotic agitation

  ➧ *Akathisia pg 640 and pg 644*

7.3.7

- **Tardive dystonia: 'Pisa syndrome'**
  This is an example of a drug-induced dystonia of delayed onset. This man leans like the Tower of Pisa, reflecting an axial dystonia of the trunk.

  ➧ *Tardive dystonia pp 642-3, 645*
  ➧ *Dystonias pp 669-70*

M7 SUMMARY

We've got to the end of module seven.

There may be either too much movement (hyperkinesia) or too little movement (hypokinesias). Additionally, there are effects on the tone (dystonias) or involuntary spasm. Importantly for neuropsychiatrist, many of these conditions are iatrogenic and care must be taken to monitor and manage treatment carefully, especially with neuroleptic drugs.

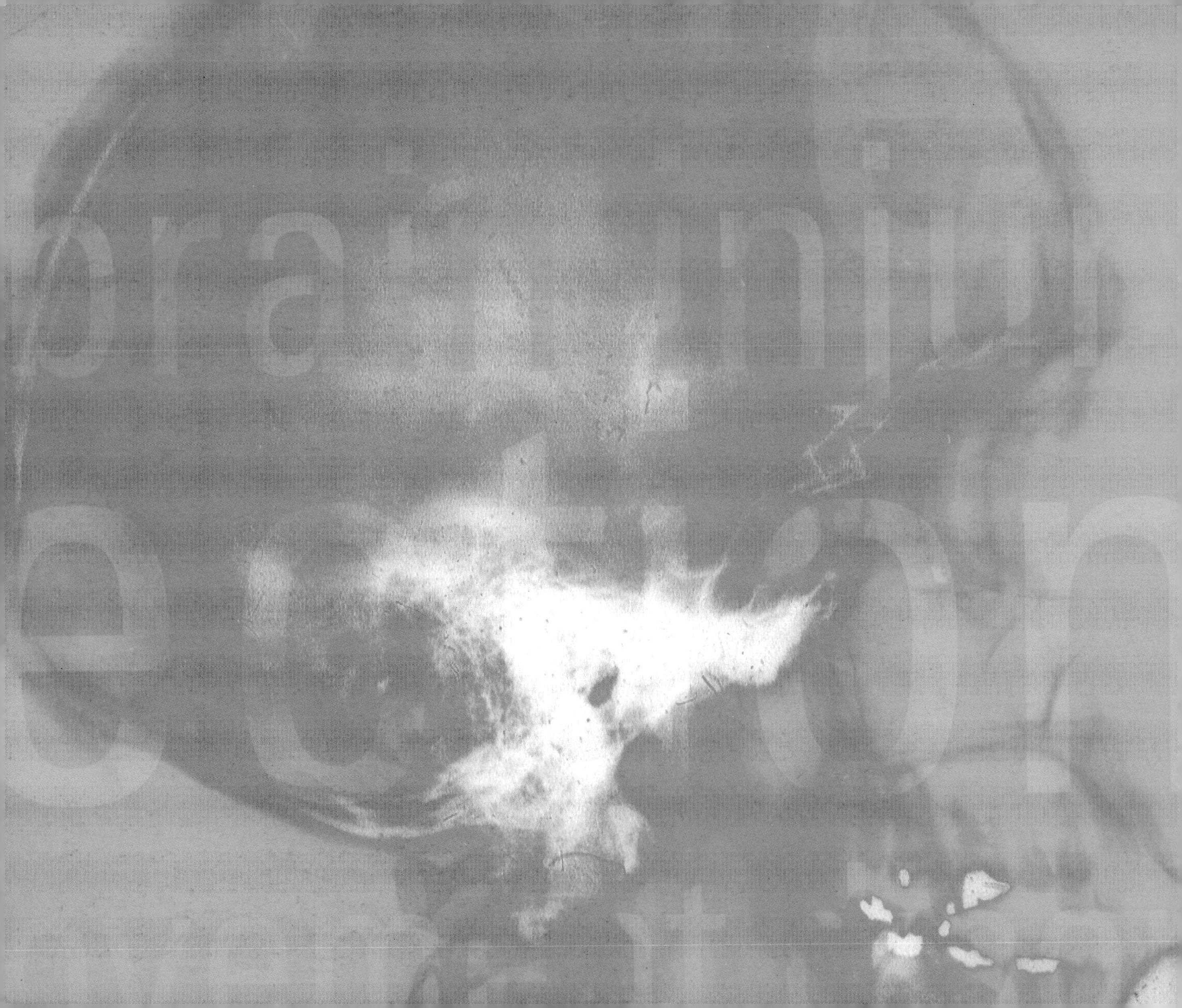